Praise for

Deborah Roffman:

"I only wish that my wife and I had this book when we were raising our children! Actually, I wish my parents had had this book too! Wise, honest, and funny, Deborah Roffman addresses all the fears and hesitations parents have about talking to their children about sexuality, puts the topic in its proper, broader context of parenting, and gives helpful advice."

—Rabbi Elliot N. Dorff, Ph.D., is Distinguished Service Professor of Philosophy at
American Jewish University and author of *Love Your Neighbor and Yourself*

"Reading this book is like sitting down with a wise, warm, and supportive best friend—she happens to be a sexuality educator—who tells you 1) what's really going on with kids and sex; 2) why this is happening; and 3) what you need to do about it. Deborah Roffman will make you feel confident that you *can* and *will* handle this crucial parenting task. Read this book. You and your kids will be glad you did."

—Steve Clem, Executive Director,
Association of Independent Schools in New England

"Deborah Roffman is one of the most enlightened thinkers in the field of sexuality education today. To truly understand what sexuality education is all about, people of all ideologies need to stop digging in their heels, and truly *listen* to what Roffman has to say."

—William J. Taverner, Editor, *American Journal of Sexuality Education*

"Deborah Roffman is our most articulate champion of sensible and wise sexuality education. I have referenced her work in conversations with my own children, and recommend her to all parents who wrestle with the question, 'So, how do I talk with my kids about sex?'"

—Michael Brosnan, Editor, *Independent School,*
National Association of Independent Schools

"Deborah Roffman has been my 'go-to' person for parents, faculty, and students when it comes to having a sane, healthy, and helpful conversation about that 'scary' subject called sexuality. The fears and awkwardness are replaced by intelligent, thoughtful commentary, and school communities are happy, relieved, and enlightened once Debbie has spent some time with them!"

—Matthew Stuart, Head of Caedmon School and
former Middle School Head at National Cathedral School

Praise for

Sex and Sensibility:

"[Roffman] talks to parents in a kind but frank tone that is bound to help them help their kids."

—Psychology Today

"[Roffman's] insights and tips are outstanding . . . highly recommended."

—Library Journal

"This book intelligently covers a crucial issue for parents."

—Publishers Weekly

"[*Sex and Sensibility*] untangles the knotted ball of yarn that we have made of the subject."

—Baltimore Sun

"A remarkably wise book. It offers a new way of thinking about sex and sexuality."

—Michael Gurian, author of The Wonder of Boys

"A really great book. . . . [Roffman's] obviously deep commitment to the sexual health of children and teenagers was touchingly powerful."

—Baltimore's Child

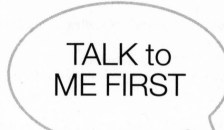

Also by
Deborah Roffman:

Sex & Sensibility

But How'd I Get in There in the First Place?

TALK to
ME FIRST

EVERYTHING YOU NEED TO KNOW
TO BECOME YOUR KIDS'
GO-TO PERSON ABOUT SEX

BY DEBORAH ROFFMAN

Da Capo

LIFE
LONG

A Member of the Perseus Books Group

Library of Congress Cataloging-in-Publication Data

Roffman, Deborah M.
    Talk to me first : everything you need to know to become your
kids' "go-to" person about sex / by Deborah Roffman. — 1st ed.
        p.   cm.
    Includes bibliographical references and index.
    ISBN 978-0-7382-1508-2 (pbk. : alk. paper) — ISBN 978-0-7382-1587-7 (e-book)
    1. Sex instruction for children. 2. Sex instruction for teenagers. 3. Sexual ethics
for teenagers. 4. Parent and child. 5. Parent and teenager. I. Title.
HQ53.R64 2012
613.9071—dc23

                                                                      2012006068

First Da Capo Press edition 2012

Published by Da Capo Press
A Member of the Perseus Books Group
www.dacapopress.com

Da Capo Press books are available at special discounts for bulk purchases in the US by corporations, institutions, and other organizations. For more information, please contact the Special Markets Department at the Perseus Books Group, 2300 Chestnut Street, Suite 200, Philadelphia, PA, 19103, or call (800) 810-4145, ext. 5000, or e-mail special.markets@ perseusbooks.com.

To
Julie Levison and Shira Wallach
Two Women of Valor

In Memoriam
Evelyn B. T. McClain

Contents

Preface

Everywhere I go, it seems, parents today are wringing their hands over the influence of media, technology, and popular culture in their kids' lives. They want to know how to deal with the pressures they and their children are facing, and how to have an equal say, at least, in shaping their children's attitudes and values, especially about sex.

If that's you, too, you've come to the right book. What I hope you'll find on every page are "ways in" to the conversations you most want to have about topics you most hold dear, with kids of all ages. Moreover, each chapter will teach you how to be a proactive nurturer around issues of sexuality, so you can stay well ahead of the media and advertising tsunami that just keeps coming and coming at American families 24/7/365.

Many things stand in the way of American parents' taking their rightful role as their children's primary go-to resources about sexuality. Expect to examine them in detail in the early chapters of the book, so it will become easier for you to take on the roles and suggestions you'll find on its pages.

Talk to Me First is also very much about this wacky American culture of ours, which *still* can't seem to decide if sex is the best thing in the world or the worst thing in the world; the most serious topic around or the most reliable fodder for joke-making from the playground to the late-night television screen; a holy sacrament or "no big deal"; the highest form of human physical and emotional intimacy, or a "quickie" between relative strangers. Our children truly are caught in the crossfire of all this confusion, struggling to make sense of these obsessive and polar opposite fixations. It's parents more than anyone who can help them find their way through the morass.

What I hope you'll discover most of all, if you haven't already, is the joyfulness to be found in educating and guiding your children around this most central and amazing part of our humanity. It's a joyfulness I've experienced in educating my own two sons and—lucky me!—in educating thousands and thousands of other people's sons and daughters in the sexuality classes and courses I've taught for more than forty years in elementary, middle, and high schools. The opportunity to spread the joy to other adults—parents and teachers I've taught and mentored over the decades at more than 250 public and private schools—has been the icing on the cake.

And so, I give you *Talk to Me First.* Enjoy!

1

Getting There
First About Sex

Meet Susie, a fourth grader who's gregarious and bright as all get out. Susie's frames of reference about the subject of sex are her older sister, her puberty education class at school, and the sexy pictures she finds online, including images of women performing oral sex on men. Susie also thinks women get pregnant by kissing.

Connor is another fourth grader in New Jersey. One day in the cafeteria line, he turns to a fourth-grade girl and asks nonchalantly, "Do you spit or swallow?" He looks entirely bewildered by the horrified expression on his teacher's face.

Mario, a pint-size fifth grader, seeming a little worried, wants to know at what age boys should start taking "male enhancement" pills, while Jasmin, his best friend, is so mortified by the whole topic of puberty she wants to hide under the desk whenever her teacher mentions the word.

And Jasmin's fifteen-year-old brother, Michael, thinks that easy access to pornography is an amazing gift to his generation. He earnestly wants to know how earlier generations got to learn about "real sex."

Welcome to the wide, wide world of "sex education" as our children experience it in the new millennium. Over the past ten-plus years, the once impermeable or at least opaque boundaries between the adult world and the world of children and teens have practically vanished. Young people now are natives in a virtual 24/7 sexuality classroom, with no guide, teacher, or parent in charge. Teens, preteens, and even young children potentially see, hear, and read it all: conversations, advertisements, movies, books, song lyrics, TV shows, texts, games, billboards, and phone and computer screens so laced with sexual imagery, language, and innuendo that many of them must conclude, at least unconsciously, that sex must be life itself, or the absolute most important thing in it.

The topic of sexuality is one of the great "equalizers" in American society. Across the United States, and in all walks of life, I find in my travels an astonishing lack of confidence and competence among adults when it comes to talking to their kids. So many otherwise capable, thoughtful, well-educated adults everywhere who are seemingly clueless about how to start even the most rudimentary of conversations! And each year, it seems, parental anxiety becomes more palpable, perhaps because with each passing year American culture becomes more noxious. In very potent ways—we'll explore these in detail in Chapter 2—the advertising, merchandizing, and entertainment industries now project imagery and messages that in some cases near totally distort who children and adolescents are and *what they need* from an accurate developmental perspective.[1] In the face of so much unhealthy competition, many parents I know feel truly at a loss. And so the cycle continues: less confidence among parents emboldening more and more aggressiveness among marketers.

But here's the very good news about parents' insecurity, even in today's world: it's so unnecessary. Like you, most parents are good parents, and plenty smart and resourceful, too. You and they handle all kinds of tricky and difficult conversations with kids all the time. But for *no good reason,* and I do mean that literally, when it comes to this particular subject even the best of minds can go to mush. And what an awful and strange feeling that is, especially when you know yourself to be and take pride in being an otherwise competent and capable adult, and a caring, willing, and responsive parent.

Mental Mush and Hairy Bears

One frustrated father I know describes these moments of mental mush as *brain lock,* similar to the experience of being tongue-tied, he says, only worse. I think he's right on.

Brain lock is an irritatingly familiar experience. For instance, almost every-one can relate to the maddening experience of your mind going blank during a test, or thinking of the perfect thing to say to your boss *right after* you leave the tense meeting in her office. This mental mushiness can emerge in virtu-ally *any* situation where you feel personally threatened, be it physical, social, emotional, and/or intellectual. Ironically, no matter how miserable or stupid it might make us feel, there is a normal physiological explanation for this sudden loss of brain power: it's a predictable and intentionally functional component of our inborn defense mechanism against danger, known to sci-entist as the "fight, flight, or freeze response."

People used to live in the wild, of course, when these physiological mech-anisms were literally lifesavers. Whenever someone spotted a perceived threat to well-being—usually a potentially dangerous person or animal—specific biological responses kicked in immediately to prepare the body to do one of the following posthaste: *run* if there was a good chance of outpacing the threatening creature, *fight* if there was a better chance of overpowering it, or, if neither plan A nor plan B was in the cards, *freeze* so as to decrease the chance of being seen (or eaten).

Problem is, we don't live in the wild today, and the kinds of threats we encounter in life are way more likely to be social, emotional, and intellectual than physical. ("I didn't know the first three answers on this quiz and I'm going to get a D and lose my scholarship and flunk out of school and I'll never get a job and my parents will kill me.") To the body, however, a threat is a threat is a threat, and its response is going to be pretty much the same *no matter the stressor*. Unfortunately, in every case, it's the extremities that are going to be oxygenated (to facilitate flight, fight, or freeze) at the ex-pense of the part of the brain that solves math problems, analyzes poetry, constructs a gorgeous sentence, turns out a clever retort, or produces a calm, brilliant response to a totally out of the blue and/or embarrassing question from a fourteen-year-old about sex. (You knew we would get back to sex, right?)

Decades ago, doctors and psychologists recognized this physiological anachronism and developed stress management and calming techniques (breathing, relaxation, etc.) to help us convince our bodies that there isn't *really* a big hairy bear out there waiting to eat us. But here's the relevant question: While the experience of blowing an important test or a crucial meeting with your boss might indeed result in scary real-life consequences, just how and why did even the thought of talking to children about sex become so intrinsically attached to the perception of danger or threat? How did it become such an automatic stressor?

I saw a television ad just the other day where two parents were arguing over who was going to give the kids "the talk." They kept sparring with each other, lobbing the dreaded conversation back and forth—you do it, no you do it—like a game of hot potato. I know this was supposed to be humorous and that a lot of people watching would easily relate, but I thought to myself, how ridiculous! I mean, we're all grown adults here, right? What *precisely* are we so afraid of?

In many American families, sexuality is the big pink elephant in the corner, *and* the big hairy bear in the back yard. Just as our bodies were built for survival in a very different time and place, our misplaced anxieties about "sex education"—often verging on nothing short of dread—were built into our culture and psyches hundreds of years ago. Though we are now launched well into the twenty-first century, American attitudes *still* are anchored in a way of life fashioned in the seventeenth. Now there's an embarrassing truth.

In fact, on January 1, 2010, I up and declared a New Decade's resolution: by 2020, families and schools in America will decide that it is probably best to raise children in the century in which they are currently living.

The year 2020, I think, is the perfect symbolic choice, since it happens to coincide with the four hundredth anniversary of the year the Puritans first came to America. Before you laugh (people like to laugh at the Puritans), and in the spirit of full disclosure, when it comes to sexuality the Puritans have been wrongly portrayed. Despite what most Americans believe, these oft-maligned ancestors were not hopelessly antisexual, or sexually repressed. In reality, they enjoyed a fundamentally healthy respect for sexuality and its place in life, and regarded sexual behavior within marriage as both a duty and a gift from God. Their ideas were not at all puritanical in the modern use of the word, which is to say they were not prudes. To the contrary, their basic beliefs mirrored the remarkably sex-positive attitudes of the ancient Hebrews, who valued the pleasure and intimacy-enhancing aspects of sexual behavior just as highly as they did procreation.

What the Puritans did disdain, however, was any kind of *public discourse* about sex, because sex was also viewed as exquisitely private. Violations of their leaders' strict taboos about public disclosure could bring severe consequences to the offender. Given the threat of public humiliation, banishment, or worse, people at the time developed a dread but rational fear of what could happen if the subject of sex "got out." But as the centuries passed, and as this and other religious and secular influences coalesced into a uniquely American brew of sexual attitudes and beliefs, this once reality-based fear morphed into a wholly irrational one, still with us today: direct and open discussion about sex isn't bad because it might be dangerous *practically* (as in, it might get you in trouble), but because it might be dangerous *intrinsically* (as in, the danger lies within the speech or the knowledge itself).

My own parents took this ominous warning very seriously. In our household knowledge about sex was kept safely tucked away in a little box in the basement, on the very top shelf in a back room, with the light out and the door tightly shut, or so it seemed. Very occasionally and with no predictability whatsoever, one of my parents would take down the box (the metaphor of Pandora's box is a perfect fit) and give my brother or me a sliver of information, or once in a while, a small nugget. Then *whoosh,* the box was gone, though the anxiety attached to its contents lingered in the house like a foreboding cloud. Even now, if I try I can conjure up that strange and, at the time, inexplicable feeling of threat.

Though my dad and mom were born in 1908 and 1914, respectively, I still see and hear evidence of modern-day "Puritan speak," as I call it, every single day in my work. A case in point: Not long ago I was asked to give a talk for parents at an elementary school. Walking into the building, I spotted a poster announcing the presentation. Well, sort of announcing it. Though the title on the poster originally read, "How to Talk with Your Children About Sex," someone had covered over the word "sex" with a half sheet of paper with three dots instead.

I glanced over at one of the parent organizers, who said, "The principal saw the poster and decided that elementary school children should not see the word 'sex' in a school building." What's a child curious about sex to do? I wondered. Go home and Google it? (Now that's something I would definitely consider intrinsically dangerous.)

By the way, the very next week I gave a talk at another elementary school very close by. Behind the refreshment table stood a father wearing a T-shirt sporting the message, "I Love My Hot Wife." I wondered if he was going to be sent to the principal's office.

If you ask them directly, parents and teachers today won't say they consciously believe that sexual knowledge is inherently bad or dangerous. But if you listen to their deepest concerns and anxieties about sexuality education, especially for the youngest of children, but often for older kids as well, there is definite unease, sometimes even a palpable sense of dread.

You definitely don't want to teach them "too much, too soon," right? But what if they're too young, or they're not "ready," or they ask *too* many questions, or—oh my God—they tell other children at school? What if those kids don't already know? What will their parents say? They'll be furious! Is it *really* okay for them to know the word "vagina"? But won't they lose their "innocence"? Yes, but if they know about it, won't they want to—you know—do it? Shouldn't you wait until they ask? For sure, you definitely don't want to tell them about contraception, because they'll assume you're giving them permission.

And there it is: just beneath the surface of all that angst is the space where the Puritans are still alive and well and speaking to us from the grave. *Beware sexual knowledge! It must be given in just the right amounts, in just the right way, by just the right person, and at the exact right moment or . . . bad things will happen!*

Because they, too, grew up in the seventeenth century, today's parents and teachers, particularly of young children, still haven't a clue about what actually *is* the right time and the right way and the right person and the right amount, so they tiptoe around the topic of sexuality gingerly at best. And many do it with a gut sense that they are being prudent and protective, even though they hardly ever can articulate what it is exactly they're so frightened of. Falsely reassured they're doing the right thing, they continue to believe their own Puritan speak and as a result miss all kinds of opportunities to "get there first." With their avoidance and delay *they only guarantee, especially in today's world, that it will be someone else* (read: peers or media) who will become their children's first, and thereby most important, sexuality educator.

So, what is there to be afraid of (nothing!), and what's the problem anyway if we keep children in the dark (plenty!)? If we're ever to throw off our puritanical heritage—the *real* one—so we can stop being afraid of all the wrong things, American families and schools need to recognize and put to rest this stunningly irrational double standard that we apply to sexual learning.

After all, as a culture we virtually (pun intended) worship knowledge about practically every other aspect of human existence. Truly, all we really need do to bring this topic into the twenty-first century is simply decide to apply the same standards to learning about sexuality—Knowledge is good! Knowledge is the cornerstone of responsibility! Knowledge is the key to a fulfilling life!—as we do all others.

Said another way, we have to stop thinking *emotionally* about this topic and start thinking *educationally.*

The very good news is that the developmentally correct benchmarks for sexual learning—what kids should know and when they should know it—are already well established by researchers and educators, and have been available for decades. (Isn't it interesting that most adults, including most educators, don't know they even exist.) It should be shocking to us that the typical American school is anywhere from three to seven years late in providing even the basics. And yet, most Americans—including parents, teachers, administrators, politicians, and policy makers—don't have the background knowledge to recognize how far off the mark schools truly are. Imagine the marching and picketing and shouting if a school district decided to postpone teaching arithmetic until the eighth grade, and then on top of that expected the students to start right away with algebra.

We Just Don't Have Another Decade to Waste

This book is for all parents who want to be certain they, too, are not afraid of the wrong things—such as providing accurate knowledge from a caring adult—and who want to become the most credible and influential resource in their children's lives about sexuality. It's for parents who want to "get there first," because that's our job, and because the default options—in particular the advertising, merchandising, and entertainment industries—become more potent in children's lives every day. And it's for parents who want to become and remain their children's primary—as in first and most important—reference points about sexuality, so that it will be *their* voice in their children's head, and *their* lens over their children's eyes, and that no matter what children hear, see, and read afterward or elsewhere about sexuality, it will be filtered through *their* "spin" as the people in the world who most have their children's best interests at heart.

After all, children always look first to the immediate adults in their lives for guidance and for framing the world in a way they can relate to and understand. They go elsewhere only when they know or sense that we are not willing to be present or available. So, why should this topic be any different? What decades of research demonstrate should be no great surprise: families who sustain this kind of connectedness around issues such as sexuality raise healthier children who make better decisions, take greater responsibility for their actions, and perhaps most important, postpone potentially risky behaviors significantly longer than peers who lack this kind of support. Knowing, in other words, leads to knowing and thinking and postponing. It's the *opposite* of dangerous.

A Promise About This Book

How freeing it is, magical really, to accept that talking forthrightly to our kids about sexuality is the *very best thing we can do* to help keep them healthy and safe. That singular realization is all we need to grab back our common sense from an ill-fated legacy that has gotten in the way of the sacred relationship between parents and children for generations and, all too often, with negative and even tragic consequences.

Many of you reading this book didn't need the last few pages to convince you that talking, talking, talking to kids is vital. You've already buried the Puritans (though it's important for everyone to understand why so many people in our communities have not, and to help bring them up to speed). You just want to know what to say and how and when to say it. You look to books like this because it's not always easy to figure that out, but only because we haven't had a lot of practice, and because most of us didn't have grown-ups in our lives who were able to demonstrate what an adult actually looks and sounds like when talking openly and confidently with a young person about sexuality. So, this book aims to provide lots of practice, and lots of modeling.

Here's the absolute promise I make to you in writing this book: even if the subject of sex sometimes makes you feel like a blubbering idiot, you will come to discover on these pages that *you are instead a wise sage* who can handle this essential topic just as capably as all others in your children's lives. Here are some specific things you will learn how to do:

- ✓ Become more "askable" and approachable about sexual topics
- ✓ Initiate conversation, even when faced with an uncomfortable or reluctant child or teen
- ✓ Invite open-ended conversations about sexual attitudes and values
- ✓ Know when clear limits and boundaries are what your children need around their social lives, and when it's time, gradually, to turn them over to themselves
- ✓ Avoid telling children and teens "too much," and most important, leaving them with too little
- ✓ Create an ongoing series of conversations about life—not sex—with your kids and make myriad connections for them about how those lessons apply to the sexual parts of life as well
- ✓ Put meaningful context around the topic of sexuality, in a world where your kids receive dozens if not hundreds of out-of-context messages each and every day
- ✓ Make these vital conversations with children and adolescents of all ages more natural, integrated, positive, and, best of all, a source of enjoyment and pride

But First, What Else Might Get in Our Way?

We Americans are susceptible and subject all the time to wildly wrong-headed ideas about sexuality education. Well-meaning but misinformed people reference and reinforce them all the time, but these ideas can shut down communication with our kids—and steal our confidence—before we even get started. Here are some of the most common culprits; once we identify and learn to give them up the whole process looks a lot more doable.

"Kids today know more than the adults"

I always joke that if my mother entertained hopes and dreams that one day I'd become a sexuality educator, she definitely never mentioned them. (She hardly ever mentioned periods either.) Like most sexuality educators around my age, there was no "career path" that brought us here. Along with many others, I became one totally by accident, in my case literally by falling into a job in a related field. When I was hired, in fact, my entire "formal" sex education had consisted of a film in the fifth grade about menstruation and deodorant and the few tidbits of information I could glean between the lines of my (abnormal) psychology text in college.

Once on the job, I learned an enormous amount very quickly by devouring everything I could get my hands on, but I freely admit that for the next ten years, at least, I was convinced I'd missed something *really* big. I lived in fear—because I didn't know what I didn't know—that one day I would expose my raw ignorance about something everyone else knew, and make a total spectacle of myself. (Mercifully, and inexplicably; I was spared.)

My insecurity was inevitable, given the entirely inadequate and haphazard way I learned about sexuality growing up. Children learn best, of course, in just the opposite manner: in a conscious, deliberate, and ever-evolving learning spiral in which teachers and parents intentionally expose them to facts and ideas that are increasingly complex and interconnected. Most adults in the United States, even today, grew up absent any kind of intentional learning spiral around the topic of sexuality, and no doubt for many of us our knowledge base is somewhat shaky, if not pathetically thin. (When I first entered the field, I could not have correctly labeled even the female reproductive parts.) It's natural, especially in today's world, where our kids are exposed to so much sexual content all the time, to feel insecure and left behind in the dust.

To all of this I say: relax! Truthfully, if you know and try to communicate information even to high school kids that's much beyond a seventh-grade level of understanding, you're trying too hard. There are really only a few basic facts about sexual health—we'll go over much of this topic later—that we need to make sure kids know and know well. Other stuff is nice or interesting to know, but not at all essential. Helping them understand which kind of information is which is our real job.

For more than three decades at my home school, I've taught a required, semester-long course for seventh graders called Human Sexuality. My course page on the school's website says, "Human Sexuality: It's Not About Sex." Culturally we focus so much on the "sex" part of sexuality, it's easy to miss the most important point of all: education about sexuality is education about life itself—and *that's* something we truly do know a great deal more about than our children *and* can feel very confident about. *Our job, really, is to teach children as much as we possibly can about how life works, and to keep pointing out all along the journey how those truths about life connect to sexuality, too.* If we're obsessed with the physical facts because of our own discomfort or anxiety, we'll inevitably end up talking about sex in mechanical and disconnected ways that will only mirror and reinforce what they see everywhere else in American popular culture.

Remember, too, that no matter how much our kids may know, they know it only on a third-, fifth-, eighth-, or twelfth-grade level. We need not let their pseudo-sophistication about grown-up subjects—which they often delight in displaying—deceive or intimidate us. Twelve-year-olds, for example, have only a dozen years of experience and the brain development of an early adolescent. One of the reasons they sometimes think (and act) as if they know everything is that in their mind, they absolutely do. They may know absolutely everything they're capable of understanding at their age about a particular subject, but their limited brainpower can't support them in imagining what else they might *not* know. If we allow ourselves to be cowed or bamboozled by any of this, we won't see who they really are and what they really need.

"I couldn't say that; I'd just be too uncomfortable"

I gave a talk in Boston recently where a woman in the back row said she was in total disbelief about my suggestions to the assembled group of parents. It wasn't that she disagreed with me, just that she didn't think she could possibly talk to her children about "it" in those ways. When I inquired what she meant by "it," she answered, "Well, you know, SEX." I asked her to speak up, but she was incapable of saying the word above a barely audible whisper. And I am not making this up.

The good-natured audience took her on as a group project. They cajoled, and joked, and prodded until finally she said "SEX" to resounding applause. I asked for other examples of words the parents didn't think they could say out loud to their kids, and out they tumbled: masturbation, testicles, clitoris, penis, vagina, erection, anus, lesbian, orgasm, and the like. Everyone got to see that these are just words, only a bunch of harmless letters of the alphabet strung together somewhat randomly. They just needed some practice to "get it."

Here's the straight-on truth: as parents we don't get to decide that we're too uncomfortable to parent. If as parents in the 1950s we had been embarrassed to say the words "polio epidemic," we would have known we would just have to get over it for the sake of our children's health. There are no free passes and no rationalizations that get us off the hook. And besides, having the courage to say, "I'm really embarrassed, and I'm going to talk about this anyway," is the best kind of modeling we can offer our kids. Doing this also teaches an important physiological fact: the vocal cords do work even when the face is red.

Almost always, whenever parents linger after a talk to ask questions, someone—almost always a woman or a gay dad—remarks, "I wish my partner/spouse would have agreed to come to this, but he says he would just be too uncomfortable to talk about sex stuff with the children." Years ago I empathized—there are indeed lots of reasons these conversations might be an even bigger challenge for dads—or offered suggestions. But now, since the default options for our kids have become so disgusting and unhealthy, I very directly encourage and even urge spouses and partners to be much more straightforward with each other about what is really a potentially harmful form of abdication. As I said, we don't rightfully get to decide that we're too uncomfortable to parent, especially not when so much is at stake.

Not only that, but discomfort connected to the topic of sexuality is really nothing more than a learned association. Truly, we weren't born uncomfortable. We absorbed it by osmosis, and what has been learned can be *un*learned by adults who are willing to step up. It's well worth it, too: for a dad to be "askable" and approachable is a *huge* gift to our sons and daughters. Besides, what children and adolescents really need to see and hear in their everyday lives are everyday adults—dads, moms, stepmoms and stepdads, guardians, foster parents, grandparents (yes, even grandparents), teachers, clergy, women, and men—talking about sexuality in sensitive, normal, and matter-of-fact ways.

Recently a fourth-grade boy told our class a story about when he learned how babies are made. He remembered being curious about this when he was six (right on developmentally, as we'll see). He'd asked his father about it, but Dad pretended not to hear him. He tried a couple more times—same nonresponse—but the fourth time was the charm. His dad just explained the basics, and that was that. Dad must have finally realized that *whenever* his son asked him to be there for him, that was exactly what he was supposed to do: be there.

"They're just not ready"

If I had a dollar for every time I've heard this one, I could endow an entire human sexuality department at my school. Usually what people mean by "not ready" is that children, especially young ones, aren't *emotionally* ready to know about sex. And, of course, they're not. That is, they're not ready or even at all interested in knowing about sex in an adult context. They aren't ready to go out and make a living, either, but they can understand the concept of money and some of the things you can do with it. In other words, they're ready for beginning concepts that later in life will help them become financially independent.

Children are intellectually or cognitively primed to learn basic concepts about sexuality—and more and more sophisticated ones later on—just as easily as any other subject. Too often adults project their own emotionality about the subject and then can't step back far enough to realize that perhaps *they* are the ones who aren't ready emotionally. To children sexuality starts out as just another new and interesting topic they enjoy thinking, wondering, and learning about. In most respects, to them it's emotionally neutral; only their brain cells need to be ready.

"My kids are too old; if I haven't told them yet, it's too late now"

If you think of your job as "teaching the kids about sex"—that is, the "facts of life" and related information—I suppose this sentiment has some merit. But truly that's the least of it. As we will come to understand it, our sexuality is a part of us that changes and develops as we do from birth onward. Children, young adolescents, high school kids, and college students (not to mention thirty-two-year-olds, forty-seven-year-olds, and seventy-year-olds) are *continually* sorting out who they are as sexual and gendered people. As parents we're never done, and it's never too late to play a role in supporting children's healthy sexual development, even if it's simply by e-mailing your kids articles you come across about sexual health, relationships, or other important topics once they're away at college or otherwise out of the house on their own.

Indeed, making the mental shift from seeing yourself as a periodic "information giver" about sex, to becoming an ongoing "nurturer" around their healthy sexual development, is central to providing kids what they most need. Even if your kids are in their late teens and there have been few conversations in the past, you can *always* have an impact if you take a deep breath and then speak straight from your heart about your hopes and concerns for their happiness and health.

"Maybe I'm just too old-fashioned"

This misconception is one that makes me especially nuts. Unless you're planning to keep your kids from dating until age eighteen, and to sit in the back of the movie theater with a flashlight when the movie starts, I would hardly call you old-fashioned.

I wonder sometimes what "history" means to kids now—life as it existed two iPods ago? (By the time this book is in its second printing, God willing, readers will be saying to themselves, "What's an iPod?") The expression "That's *so* yesterday!" can almost be taken literally today, given the dizzying rate of change with respect to technology and media. I worry that to kids "old" has come to mean useless and irrelevant, something that no longer works or applies, and that "new" is automatically better than what's "not new."

As parents, many adults I know feel "old," as in superfluous and even obsolete, well before their time. They view themselves almost like adjuncts in their children's lives instead of central or supporting characters, and though that's an understandable reaction in the context of today's world, it's entirely misguided. They've forgotten that *the more some things change in children's lives, the more other things need to stay exactly the same.* Remaining an engaged and involved parent is not old-fashioned—it's not about "fashion" at all. It's essential. There's no substitute for it, and whenever we're feeling on the outside looking in, it's usually because of something we're doing, or not doing, as parents and not that our kids don't need us.

As I listen to parents talk about what they want for their children as emerging sexual people, there's nothing old-fashioned there either. The pop culture standard of "anything goes" when it comes to sex isn't "new-fashioned"; it's no standard at all. Heaven help us all when having standards in life becomes passé. Though it may be much trickier today to compete with the outside influences in children's lives, it just means we have to work harder and smarter. Expect many suggestions on how to do this in the chapters to come.

"I'm not that liberal"

In case you've not noticed, almost everything about sexuality—gay rights, abortion, sex education, emergency contraception for younger teens, stem cell research, health coverage for contraception, etc.—is highly politicized in the United States. With the country seemingly polarized about so many issues today, and the news cycle awash in "controversies" designed to keep us interested 24/7, perennial hot-button topics such as sexuality are framed almost exclusively in political terms or reduced to either/or dichotomies.

One outcome has been the unfortunate conflation of politics and parenting around sexuality, and a slew of misleading and unhelpful stereotypes: liberal parents are "open" with their kids, while conservative parents hold "traditional values." Liberals buy their kids condoms; conservatives say "abstinence only until marriage." Gay is okay; gay is bad. Sex education belongs in schools; no, only in the home. You would think there was no middle ground to be found, only opposite and opposing camps.

In reality, of course, there are amazing and wonderful parents on both sides of the aisle. Very "open" ones on the Right, and deeply religious ones on the Left. There are "permissive" Republican parents, and strict Democratic ones. There are lesbian and gay parents across the spectrum, as well as parents for and against abortion rights. And all of them are raising *children,* who have or need no political or party affiliation at all, just parents—and communities—who see them and their needs through a developmental (not political) lens and who don't confuse politics and parenting.

Little-Box Thinking About Sex and Sexuality

If you think about it, all these considerations do serve a purpose: they give adults permission—justification, even—for putting off conversations about sexuality indefinitely. How convenient, and all the more reason to keep re-examining our common nonsense about sexuality education.

Decades ago it occurred to me that American society suffers from a curious kind of sexual-learning disability. Many (really, really smart) people simply don't know how to think about these topics in deep or nuanced ways; it's as if there's a hole in their brain—a virtual disconnect in the circuitry—between the topic of sexuality and what they know and can apply so effortlessly to other parts of life. Truthfully, we can look back to the Puritans' real legacy in American society to explain this, too: if you're not allowed to speak about something freely or to argue about it in the public square, or read or write about it, you can't learn to ask good questions, do independent research, think critically, and grow intellectually. (Someone in Congress was recently criticized for saying the word "uterus" on floor of the Senate. How do you debate something you can't even mention?) And because the majority of American schools today still tag sexual topics as being "off limits," I most fear we continue to groom new generations of grown-ups who will be stuck in the mud, too.

Getting Americans "unstuck" isn't as hard as it may sound. Simply challenging some of our basic assumptions about sexuality, and how we talk about it, works wonders on reconnecting what we already know about life to this subject, too.

Really Silly Stereotypes Like "the Talk"

Many Americans cling like Velcro to the image of the dreaded "Sit down—I'm going to let the cat out of the bag now" sex talk. During talks I give, everyone nods knowingly at the suggestion that, of course, the process is so much more complicated than a one-shot sit-down. But five minutes later, someone will impatiently ask, "Yes, but *exactly how and when* should I tell them about 'it'?" As we'll see in every chapter of this book, there is no "it."

When parents think they've finally spilled the beans, they often experience a genuine sense of accomplishment and a false sense of completion. Because the words and concepts may have been hard for them to say or explain, they may conclude they've done the hard part. (Once again, out of their own "stuff," they're confusing their needs with their child's reality.) Truthfully, saying all those uncomfortable words is the really easy part. Maybe they've explained the basic concept of sexual intercourse—as in, the physical juxtaposition of two particular body parts—but they've not in any way taught their child about "sex," because they've communicated little if anything about the experience or meaning of sexual behavior in people's lives, or how best to think about or understand it. Creating meaning and context around sexuality is the real challenge. Accomplishing that will take dozens and dozens of talks.

Missing the Forest for the Tree

People most often think that talking to children about sexuality means, literally, talking to children about sex. Here's the Pacific Northwest forest we miss for that tree: human sexuality is without a doubt the richest, deepest, and broadest subject there is. It's related to *virtually everything* in the world that connects meaningfully with matters of sex, gender, and reproduction. And if you think about it, that is practically everything in the world. After all, sexuality is the central life force. Why wouldn't it be connected to everything?

So, talking about sexuality also means talking about history, the arts, literature, and virtually all of the sciences; communication, relationships, family, and social networking; current events, technology, politics, government, religion, economics, media, business, and advertising; law, medicine, pharmacy, sociology, anthropology, and psychology. And that's not an exhaustive list by any means; even the most embarrassed parent, who would rather die than talk to their kids in detail about sex, can find lots of dinner-table conversation in that mix. As I've said, talking to your kids about sexuality is talking to them about life.

There's also the problem of how narrowly we define the word "sex" itself in American culture. Almost universally, Americans make use of the word "sex"—in thought, speech, and written word—as shorthand for vaginal intercourse. That's the equivalent of using the word "vegetable" as shorthand for "celery." Not only would we linguistically wipe out the entire vegetable department (except for the celery), we would have no language for talking or even thinking about peas, carrots, or broccoli. (That last example might actually make a lot of people, including my husband, pretty happy.) And then we would wonder why kids don't think string beans are *real* vegetables (or that oral sex is *real* sex, if you follow my culinary drift).

Moreover, what exactly does this shorthand definition of sex—as equivalent to vaginal intercourse—say to and about gay people? They don't exist? They don't count? They don't have sex? Oh, what confusion we sow.

Mushy Thinking About Values

The word "values" has the opposite problem: it's used to mean so many different things to so many different people it has practically no meaning at all. The trick in talking lucidly and persuasively with kids about the values you hold dear is first to stop, think, and identify the *kind of value* you want to talk about: personal, family, community, relationship, religious, moral, ethical, sexual, parental, etc. You'll be amazed at how much easier those conversations go once you can articulate with that kind of clarity. As we'll see, it's the most effective tool you have for competing with the barrage of value-laden messages your children take in every single day from the world around them.

Not "Getting" What Our Job Really Is

Someone I know once summed up what most sex education in the United States is about pretty accurately: the body parts you have, what they can do, the ways they can get you in trouble, and how to keep that from happening!

Though the emphasis on problems and prevention is certainly understandable—there are some pretty scary things out there for our kids—it exposes once again how snugly we're wedged as a culture into small-box thinking. First of all, there's no real humanity in that approach; it suggests, and kids often think this is exactly what we're suggesting, that sexuality is mostly about mechanics and body parts, not the people attached to them. People bring *all* of themselves—their whole history, their gender, their emotions, values, thoughts, needs, vulnerabilities, strengths, ideals, desires, hopes, and dreams—into every experience in life, including sexual ones. What's more, focusing on "problems" and their prevention is a fundamentally negative way of framing the whole subject to begin with.

The bottom line: the very best sexuality education at home and in schools is not about prevention, but about *creation*. Its purpose is to teach young people how to create for themselves enjoyable, caring, and responsible sexual lives. That's the key to healthy development, and also to your becoming your children's most trusted "go-to" person. When young people know that we care most about their long-term well-being—not just keeping them out of trouble—they see us as trusted guides they can come to time and time again.

Either/Or Thinking About Families and Schools

Many public discussions about "sex education" are based on a faulty notion that can prompt misleading debate and, sometimes, unnecessary rancor over the question of who should teach "it": families *or* schools. In truth, of course, there is no "it"—no box or certain quantity of information that one or the other turns over at just the right moment—since the real goal is the ongoing process of supporting children's and adolescents' healthy sexual development. That's a big job, and there's plenty that both families and schools, as the two primary nurturing institutions in children's lives who already share enormous responsibilities, can actively contribute.

The best approach is for families and schools to see themselves *in partnership,* with each playing the role best suited to their unique characteristics. For example, schools can offer ongoing, formal instruction in a planned sequenced way, while parents can engage in an endless supply of spontaneous teachable moments that family life inevitably affords. Schools can support core values—such as respect, responsibility, honesty, and compassion—right alongside parents, but parents have an additional job that schools can't begin to touch: only a parent can tell a child what she or he personally values around sexuality and all of life's other vital issues *as that child's parent.* Our roles, families and schools, can be mutually supportive in a variety of ways, but they are not interchangeable. Just because one or the other is "teaching it" doesn't let the other partner off the hook in any way.

Paying Attention to the Wrong Things

I began writing this book in the back of my mind in the aftermath of Super Bowl XXXVIII, of "wardrobe malfunction" fame. (I sat down to write my first book, *Sex and Sensibility,* a month into the Clinton-Lewinsky debacle; I'd been waiting and wishing for ages for an opening to get Americans seriously engaged in the "What is sex?" conversation, and suddenly there it was.) What grabbed me about the Justin Timberlake/Janet Jackson incident, and the swift and certain condemnation that followed, was the focus of the outrage. Almost everyone, it seemed, fixated on what appeared to be an exposed nipple, while hardly anyone even mentioned the hand that exposed it.

Everyone has nipples, right? We've *all* seen them, right? Even children have seen them. How is that even in the same ballpark as someone having the audacity and crassness to portray sexual assault—in any form—as "entertainment"? How did people miss that, and how did they end up paying attention to the wrong thing?

What a sad and lost opportunity, I thought at the time. Adults everywhere might have used the incident to teach any number of lessons about junk culture and the unhealthy attitudes and values it projects, and about the importance of respecting other people's boundaries at all times. And what a stark example of how much our feigned prudery in the United States has cost us. The most that many parents could think to do was stand in front of the TV so their kids couldn't see.

When it comes to sex, as I've said, Americans often can't see the forest for the tree. That is to say, when something explicitly sexual enters the picture, we have trouble seeing anything beyond it. What's beyond the sexual content is the *human context* in which sexuality unfolds, and that's what our kids need most of all for us to notice and talk to them about as often, and as deeply, as possible. In today's world especially they need us to keep stepping back far enough to see—and help them process—the whole forest. I hope you'll find that all-important step back on every page of *Talk to Me First,* too.

A Big Secret, and Where We Go from Here

Here's the best-kept secret about doing a fine job with this subject with your kids: there *is* no secret! That's because good parenting is good parenting is good parenting is good parenting. What I hope you'll discover in this book is that everything you already know about being a good parent applies equally to sexuality. You may think of sexuality as different, for all the reasons laid out in this chapter, but really it's exactly the same.

Count on this book to provide eight things that will help you bring everything you already know about good parenting to the sexual aspects of your children's development:

1. A new and empowering way of understanding children's sexual development, from birth through adolescence, and a blueprint for nurturing healthy sexuality at each developmental stage
2. A secure grasp of the information children and teens most need and want to know about sexuality, and pointers on how to deliver it
3. Help in clarifying your personal beliefs and values, and strategies for imparting them
4. Ways to help children and teenagers understand the importance of respecting sexual limits and boundaries, and the connection between sex and intimacy
5. Approaches for supporting your children in making healthy sexual decisions, and postponing premature involvement in sexual activities
6. An understanding of how gender impacts sexual decision-making, and how parents can positively influence how boys and girls view themselves and each other
7. Ideas for working with other parents, and with your children's schools, so we all can work together to support healthy sexual development
8. Insight into the negative cultural forces in children's lives that work against our best efforts, and ways to diminish their impact

We'll jump right into number eight in the very next chapter. The better you understand the "upside-down world" marketers and others work so hard to create, the better you'll make use of the very practical material in the rest of the book to help minimize its impact.

How to Use This Book

Talk to Me First in many ways is a departure from traditional books on "talking to the kids about sex." It's not so much a book about sex at all, but about children of all ages and their special relationship with the adult nurturers in their lives. That relationship, not sex, will be at the center of every page you'll read. In my experience, it's when parents get a really firm handle on *that,* the topic of sexuality—with some extra help to start as needed—takes care of itself. Really!

Lots of times readers pick up a book like this and flip through it for guidance about a particular issue or topic—sort of like my students do when I hand out a text (except in this book, sorry, there are no diagrams). I hope you'll find specific help for any immediate questions or concerns in the index or appendix. But as a general rule, my advice is to sit back and relax and read it straight through, since the concepts in each chapter really do build on themselves. That way you'll get the really big picture, along with a new mindset about this topic and a personal philosophy about raising sexually healthy kids—all of which I hope will be empowering, not simply helpful.

Some final words about the age of your kids: this book is written for parents of children from zero to eighteen, and even beyond. I've woven together examples from different age groups throughout each chapter, with a particular purpose in mind. Years of experience with children, adolescents, and their parents have taught me a startling truth: every child at every stage of development shares the same core developmental needs (and there are only five of them). The mixture of examples is meant to illuminate that notion, and to remind you that regardless of the timing, circumstance, or issue, your roles as a parent are constant. If you take that message to heart, you'll always know how to approach this topic, or any topic, with your kids.

For those of you with young children, I hope the information about kids older than yours will help you develop a vision and a plan for the future. If your children are older, information about earlier stages may well help you better understand who they are today, what they may have missed along the way, and how best to bring them up to speed.

You'll notice, too, that the content and examples later in the book trend somewhat toward older children and adolescents. That's because these chapters focus on what young people need as they begin to make more and more independent decisions about their social and sexual lives. For those of you raising younger kids, those chapters will help you know how to lay a foundation *now* for *then.*

2

Raising Children in a World Gone Upside Down

I n my grandmother's day, age was a fixed and finite concept. When Ida was sixty, she and everyone else her age were unquestionably "old." I can still picture her sitting on our shaded front porch for much of the afternoon "resting." At sixty my mother wasn't exactly old, but she was already retired and definitely a senior citizen.

Today, when the pace of technological and societal change makes even yesterday feel like history—and indefinite longevity an expectation—time and age seem astonishingly fluid. The perception that sixty is the new fifty, fifty the new forty, and so on seems logical and right. In fact, the day I announced in the faculty room that it was my sixtieth birthday, someone remarked, "No worries. Don't you know sixty is the *new 40*?"

How about that! I turned sixty and gained twenty years all in one morning.

So why, then, do things seem to be going in the opposite direction for our children? If thirty is the new twenty, how come, according to a *USA*

Today cover story, "Ten Is the New Fifteen"?[1] And if that's true, what does that make your five-year-old, or your fifteen-year-old? If everyone at every other stage of development is gaining time, why are children and adolescents—for whom ample time to grow up is not a luxury but a developmental imperative—losing it?

The cultural paradox is so mind-boggling it's necessary to look outside normal reason and logic—and back at American cultural history—to solve it. Unlike the life-affirming transformations for older generations, this escalating "adultification" of children and adolescents is in no way rational, healthy, or the natural course of events. To the contrary, as we'll see, it's the invention of an advertising-entertainment-merchandising industry run amok. In many ways it has literally turned the world that children used to know upside down, and it has also confused and miseducated an awful lot of parents and other adults about what children and teenagers need from the grown-ups in their lives. Knowing how to recognize and get ahead of these unhealthy distortions—the purpose of this chapter—is essential to "getting there first" and to strengthening your voice and influence as your children's primary sexuality educator.

Vanishing Boundaries in Every Direction

The vanishing boundaries between the child and adult worlds are emblematic of any number of changing norms, boundaries, and expectations in American culture:

- The notion of sex as personal and private, the very attributes that imbue it with meaning, is contradicted everywhere in popular culture—music, movies, television, video games, clothing, language, and of course the Internet. What used to be considered private and intimate is now broadcast crassly and ubiquitously.
- It's "okay" now to dress little girls in provocative clothing, buy "loungerie" for four-year-olds, facials for five-year-olds, iPhones for six-year-olds, padded bras for eight-year-olds, and Botox injections for fourteen-year-olds.

- ✓ Oral sex, thought of not so long ago by many people as even *more* intimate than sexual intercourse, is depicted as no big deal, and not particularly intimate either.
- ✓ The word "pimp" is now a compliment to a boy, and girls, who insist their choice of language doesn't mean a thing, nonchalantly call one another sluts, 'hos, and bitches.
- ✓ The advertising, merchandising, and entertainment industries unashamedly pimp men's and women's bodies to hawk everything from floor tiles, stereo amplifiers, and tuna fish to laundry detergent, breakfast cereal, and hip and back surgery. (I have the ads to prove it!)
- ✓ Pornography, previously found on the outskirts of town, or at least in the back room of the video store, is now on our children's computers and in their bedrooms; some teenagers are even making their own.
- ✓ Though women used to object to being reduced to sexual objects, many teenage girls and even women in the workplace now deliberately invite it.[2]
- ✓ Even many elementary schoolkids now use sexually explicit language whenever and wherever they please, with little or no thought to editing their words.

How did we get here? How did the relatively sane world we used to know and count on turn into a twenty-first-century Alice's Wonderland, where suddenly up is down, down is up, yet life goes on as "normal"? Why has this been allowed to happen, and what is the toll on our children? And most important, how do we turn it around?

A Look Back

The forces at work in shaping this topsy-turvy state of affairs have been decades in the making. As someone who spent her childhood in the '50s and junior high, high school, and college years in the '60s, and who has been a sexuality educator practically ever since, I've been watching them unfold from a singularly unique perch.

Over the years I've heard plenty of partisan declarations about whom or what to fault for these disturbing changes—it's the parents, the kids, the media, sex education, the '60s, the '70s—and highly politicized ones: It's the liberals! The so-called sexual revolution (in reality, more a revolt than a revolution; more on that later), and the ever-cascading breakdown in traditional and moral values it supposedly unleashed, tends to get the most play by politicians and pundits. (Even the Catholic Church recently blamed it for the misbehavior of its priests.)[3] But I'm convinced the "experts" and analysts are pointing their fingers at the wrong decades, and the wrong set of causes.

How AIDS Changed Everything

Despite the legendary upheavals of the 1960s, it's important to know that in reality mainstream America remained steadfastly buttoned-up about sexual matters well into the 1980s. For sure, there was lots of sexual innuendo in entertainment venues, advertisements, and the like, but the nation's official sources of information—newspapers, news magazines, and TV news programming—near totally refrained from printing or broadcasting any explicit sexual terms at all, whether slang or proper, even when attempting to address serious health and safety issues. Hard to believe, perhaps, but true.

The first cases of AIDS were identified in the United States in 1981. Miraculously, a short two years later, doctors and researchers had pieced together all the information the public needed to protect itself. They knew conclusively how people got, didn't get, and most important, how they could *avoid* getting, this horrible disease for which there was no cure and little or nothing in the way of treatment. If ever there was a time to stop the epidemic in its tracks, this was it. It was a breathtaking advance.

There was a hitch. Explaining HIV transmission and prevention adequately meant naming practically every verboten word or phrase on the list—penis, vaginal lubrication, oral sex, anal sex, condom, semen, ejaculation, homosexual, "gay sex," and so on. Tragically, the moment and the opportunity were lost to old-fashioned prudery and adherence to convention. I remember watching in dismay as health officials concocted and promulgated the great-grandmother of all euphemisms: "Listen up now. Just don't share bodily fluids!" Even today, my students still quote this worse than useless cliché.

Things did get better. As the disease spread and began to affect a broader cross section of the population—tragically, another significant reason for public- and private-sector inaction was bigotry and denial, because the illness was initially characterized as a "gay" disease—taboos gradually lifted. News anchors and print reporters began to give voice to people's fears, faces to those who were suffering, and crucial information to the public. One by one, the forbidden words came out of the closet, as broadcasters and editors endorsed the use of increasingly detailed and explicit information in the service of prevention. I remember sitting aghast in front of the television one morning as US Surgeon General C. Everett Koop calmly demonstrated the proper application of a latex condom, using a plastic penile model, no less. By the end of the decade, almost all sixth graders who came into my classes—twelve-year-olds are always my most reliable barometer for reading cultural change—were already familiar with words such as "monogamy" (though, in classic sixth-grade form, some mispronounced it as "mahogany").

The United States, it seemed, had finally begun to wake up—and grow up. Gradually I began to hear sexual health–related terms spoken in normal, unembarrassed tones in everyday conversation. One of the most astonishing was the matter-of-fact exchange I overheard between my husband's Uncle Leonard and another man about an article in the morning paper on "condom testing by the government." (No, it's not what you think. Really. They use machines.) They also shared a chuckle over the recently announced and far from subtle brand name of the first "large"-size condom: Magnum. To fully appreciate the gravity of the exchange, you have to understand that prior to the late 1980s hardly anybody *ever* said the word condom in "polite" company—it was then still connected most frequently with prostitution and "VD"—and this particular conversation took place between two *seventy-somethings* at a formal wedding reception.

I almost felt the earth shake. *Eureka!* I thought. *We are about to raise the first American generation of sexually literate young people, who will have what they need—comfort, awareness, knowledge—to manage and enjoy their sexuality throughout their lives in safe, healthy, and fulfilling ways.* Though there is nothing good to say about AIDS the disease, here, hopefully, was a very positive outcome of having to cope with it.

In the early 1990s, however, I detected a slight, then remarkably brazen, shift of an entirely different kind. What I hadn't thought of was that, of course, the advertising, entertainment, and merchandising industries were also watching closely. At some point, I imagine, they must have reached a collective epiphany: "Oh! This new openness about HIV has made it safe for us to be way more explicit about sex, too." As marketers set out methodically to push the proverbial envelope on explicit sexual language, references, and imagery in ways they'd not dared to before, I watched as the nation's newfound permission to educate morphed into the media's self-appointed license to titillate. At the same time, ironically, the hope for a more comprehensive approach to sexuality education fizzled, as the abstinence-only movement gained steam and many school-based programs became even more restrictive than before the epidemic.

Where It All Started

I noticed the transformation first in the women's fashion industry. To be able to see subtle and eventually more dramatic changes in print advertisements, you really have to follow them closely, both in the aggregate and over time—something I get to do routinely since my students bring me fresh batches of ads every semester. As I was perusing bunches of them in the early '90s, it became obvious that a bizarrely paradoxical shift was in the works. More and more, I realized, women's fashion seemed no longer about getting dressed, but about getting undressed. "Clothing" began to resemble what women used to wear *under* their clothing, as the new subtext in marketing images seemed to proclaim, "Underwear is the new outerwear!" (Could a Victoria's Secret lingerie "fashion show" be far behind?)

Eventually the necessity for wearing underwear—or for that matter, wearing anything—seemed to vanish altogether. Soon enough it was a common experience to flip the page in almost any magazine and find yourself confronted by fashion models portrayed in all manner of public places engaged in all manner of activities—strolling down streets, posing on mountain tops, carousing in restaurants, lounging by the pool, parading through shopping malls, etc.—while practically, or entirely, au naturel.

I noticed, too, that the pace at which marketers poked at the public's tolerance for vanishing boundaries was calibrated ever so shrewdly, just swiftly enough so that within any four- to six-month period there were perceptible shifts, but not so precipitously as to risk creating a "gasp" factor. I remember one Labor Day weekend back-to-school sale when a high-profile national department store goofed on this big time in a television ad. It opened with a teenage girl clad in a belly shirt and low-rise jeans approvingly checking herself out in the mirror. Her mom soon walked in, took one quick judgmental look, shook her head, and self-righteously proclaimed, "You are not going to school dressed like *that,* young lady!" I simply could not believe my eyes at what happened next. The woman actually went over to the daughter, yanked her pants down even farther, and said, "Now you're ready."

The ad was history before people even gassed up for the weekend.

Soon enough, other retailers got in on the act; if women didn't have to wear clothing in clothing ads, why wear clothing in *any* ads? Naked women (and some men) began popping up in ads selling everything from soup to nuts. (I haven't actually seen a sexy ad for either soup or nuts, but you should see the tuna fish ad I have.) A series of ceramic tile ads really caught my eye: "You won't believe our body of work," the text claimed. And indeed, there was a woman's body, naked except for two diamond-shaped backsplash tiles, dangling in front of each breast from a sexy lace shoulder strap. I wondered if the company's tiles came in sizes 6×6 and 12×12, or 36B and 38D.

Throughout the 1990s and into the 2000s there was hardly a whimper of protest as long-established boundaries in print ads were crossed again and again, even when they began to resemble what we used to think of in the United States as soft porn. One year around the winter holidays my husband and I were at the Metropolitan Opera. I was gawking incredulously at the ads in the playbill when I spotted one for a popular liqueur. The caption read, "Let it flow, let it flow, let it flow," over an image of liquid being poured into the center of a punch bowl. Always suspicious, I scrutinized more closely and realized that the outline of the bowl and the ripples in the middle were configured in the exact same form and proportions as an *anatomically correct vulva* (quite impressive, actually), including inner labia, outer labia, vaginal opening, and a perfectly placed and shaped clitoris. And see if you can guess where the long stream of liqueur was entering the "bowl."

Amazed, I started giving my students a new media literacy assignment: bring in an ad that uses a sexual double entendre to sell a product that has virtually nothing to do with sex. Back then it wasn't so easy, but some of the ads were actually pretty clever, if not downright cute. Two of my favorites: "The Joy of Sox"—playing on Alex Comfort's best seller, *The Joy of Sex*— sporting an array of very friendly-looking socks dangling from a warm and cozy hearth, and an Xbox ad flaunting sperm-shaped game controllers, with the tag line, "70 games, with more being conceived every day." Eventually, though, hard-core replaced cute as marketers, having gingerly crossed the initial barrier without recourse, no longer felt the need to legitimize a random sexual reference with a likeable play on words. One of my first clues was an advertisement for a stereo amplifier (brought to me by a savvy seventh grader) displaying two anorexic, drugged-looking, slave-outfitted women standing on either side of an emotionless muscle man straddling a sub-woofer, with the catchy slogan "Just plug it in and turn it on."

Today, name a product, any product, and some marketer has or someday will find a way to link it linguistically to sex. Experiencing dropped calls, or "Connectile Dysfunction"? Switch to Sprint. "Wouldn't you like to be inside me?" Become an organ donor. (Nonprofits have gotten into the act, too.) How to "respect yourself in the morning"? Eat Nutri-Grain Muffin Bars. The image for this one was a woman wearing nothing but long black boots and a delicious-looking upside-down iced banana muffin, which covered her from just underneath her arms and rounded out at the hips like a cute little muffin tutu. And who says advertisers don't take women seriously.

See if you can guess the product paired with this provocation: "I'm a Stripper." I'm sure that Breathe Right Nasal Strips leaped immediately to your mind. After all, beating the zzz's or clearing up those stuffy nasal passageways is as sexy as it gets, right?

A Sexualized Culture

So, really, what's my point? Big deal—advertisers use sex because sex sells. And certainly marketers have been using sexual allure to sell products ever since someone got the bright idea to drape a sexy-looking woman over the hood of a car (if not long before). And why focus on print advertisements from the 1990s, when network TV, cable and radio stations, magazines, movies, song lyrics, live stage performances—not to mention the Internet—have pushed all the limits, too?

Fair enough. But I contend that it's those uncontested advertisements in the 1990s and 2000s that set the stage for all the rest to seep into American life, and eventually into our children's lives. Somewhere during the 1990s, I sensed that the sheer volume and pervasiveness of sexual content—the number of sexual acts, references, and innuendos on network television alone tripled during the decade—reached a critical mass. Sexuality and sexiness, once ensconced primarily in people's personal lives, had become an inescapable intrusion into everyday living.

I remember the evening I really got it. I had just checked into a hotel in a northeastern city. It was 11 p.m. and I wanted to catch the late evening news on a local affiliate. I switched on channel 2, then channels 3, 4, and 5, until I found what I was looking for. But then I went right back to channel 4 to see if there was something wrong with my eyesight. No, I discovered, I'd seen exactly what I thought: a full-grown elephant nuzzling the vulva of a semi-naked woman lying on the ground before him with the end of his trunk. Like I said, an inescapable intrusion into everyday living. I was looking for a weather report and got bestiality instead.

It was in 1998 that juniors and seniors in my classrooms began reporting that they simply did not recognize themselves in the social experiences of their middle school–age siblings. Incredulous that a mini–generation gap somehow had crept between them in such a short time, they remarked constantly, "*We* weren't into *that*," or "We didn't know *anything* about this," or "We never even heard *that* kind of language," or "I never even *thought* about that at their age." I'm still hearing older teens speak that way about younger ones; in some ways the gap looms even larger now as the role technology plays in children's lives constantly expands and reinvents itself.

Today I'm hardly surprised by stories teachers and parents tell me about the sexually charged language and behavior even of elementary school children, given their constant exposure to a ubiquitously sexualized world. Just recently, one fifth grader in my class wanted to know how a woman could have sex with more than one man in more than one opening, and another asked, "What's 'S and M'?"

We have to keep in mind, always, that children and many adolescents still are apt to take most things at literal or face value. They don't yet have near the experience or cognitive sophistication necessary to contextualize the potent messages about sexuality they hear and see every day. Remember all of those "Isn't it time you thought about enlarging your penis?" e-mails we all used to get? Though you and I probably made a face, pressed delete, and moved on, a pre-teenage boy would be just as likely to say to himself, "Gee, I didn't know I had to worry about that!" (I once got an e-mail that boasted, "*Last chance* to enlarge your penis!" I'll admit I felt I should forward it to both of my sons, just in case.)

The sexually tinged words and images in front of our children are slick, eye-catching, and ever moving, like a kaleidoscope. In a flash, children look, hear, draw conclusions and file them away, and then repeat the process again and again, with each new inference built haphazardly on top of the last one. Eventually—if there are no adults right next to them interpreting what they see and hear—the images, words, and inferences coalesce over time to shape a misleading if not totally distorted worldview about the place and meaning of sex in people's lives. What each of them needs is their own personal cultural interpreter (that would be you!) who makes a point of looking at and listening to the world through their children's eyes and ears, stopping along the way to clarify, correct, and contextualize.[4] Much more on that in coming chapter.

What's a "Tween"?

By virtue of growing up in America, young people today simply can't avoid exposure to highly sensationalized and sexualized adult-oriented messages; it now just comes with the territory. But there's another development—one much more calculated and targeted—to explain the blurring of boundaries that once reliably separated the world of children from the world of adults: the invention and cultivation, since the mid- to late 1990s, of the market niche known as "tweens."

Like the bug zapper in my cousin's backyard that sizzles every time it fries another unsuspecting critter, part of my brain goes "*bzzt*" every time someone uses the word "tween" as if it represents a bona fide developmental stage.

In reality, "tween" is a wholly manufactured-out-of-thin-air marketing concept that lumps together—check this out—all eight- to fourteen-year-olds, as if everyone in this age group shares the same characteristics, needs, maturity, and interests.

If you know anything at all about eight-year-olds and fourteen-year-olds, you've got to be thinking, "Huh?" And yet, the invention of "tweens," and the mass marketing of thousands and thousands of products for and to them, has been wildly successful, now to the tune of $43 billion a year. The end result, I fear, has been a distortion in the minds of many children as well as adults about the nature of children and childhood itself.

The first time I personally saw the word "tween" was on the cover of *Newsweek* magazine in October 1999.[5] It appeared over the image of two self-assured and wholesome but hip-looking twelve-year-olds, both sporting brand-name clothes and designer sneakers. The lead article, "The Truth About Tweens," described a brand-new and different generation of kids about to enter the new millennium, "a generation stuck on fast forward," composed of youngsters—for example, precocious young girls all dolled up in sexy lingerie and provocative makeup and their tough-guy-swaggering macho counterparts—in a race to adulthood. Immersed in a sex-drenched media fantasy world, surrounded by an equally driven and pressured peer group, and engaged in a prematurely grown-up social life, these kids, the article advised, were in a "fearsome hurry to grow up."

Why are these kids so grown up so soon? the writers pondered. *Why are they so "preternaturally frantic"?* In part, the story argued, they are responding to the frightening and violent world around them, where events such as the Columbine massacre (which had occurred just a year before), high-profile stories about predators and kidnappers, and ubiquitous images of abducted children on milk cartons had stolen their innocence and their confidence that adults could be counted on to keep them safe. Moreover, dynamics at home—nearly half were children of divorce and more than 75 percent of their mothers were in the workforce—were causing them to have to shoulder many burdens beyond their years. "Too old for baby sitters and often alone in the afternoons with only cartoons or the computer for company," they were being forced into premature independence. In addition, the signs of puberty were beginning earlier for these kids, due to better health care and nutrition, so their own physical development conspired as well to reinforce a perfect storm of internal and external pressures to be and act more grown-up.

Not surprisingly, the article reported, researchers were beginning to discover among "tweens" and/or older teens higher rates of drinking, sexual intercourse, experimentation with oral sex, and obsessions with dieting and looks, as kids—feeling like little adults themselves—began copying what they saw in adult movies and on the Internet.

To all of this I say: Puhleeze! Give me a break.

What a tidy little package: a whole generation being turned on its ear by milk cartons, working mothers (gasp), and their own too-well-nourished pituitary glands. Though for sure the world has changed, and things are different and tough in a lot of ways for kids and families, I'm not sure how any of this explains, for example, why girls might dress in sexy lingerie and experiment with oral sex. (Heck, my mother lived through the Great Depression without doing either, I'm almost certain.) Though, I hope, fundamentally well intentioned in my book, this very first nationally published treatise on "tweens" provided way more in the way of justification than edification about a "new" developmental stage that doesn't actually exist.

Canceling Childhood

Marketers have done such a remarkable job snowing the American public about kids they cleverly call "tweens" that many people believe it to be an authentic psychological term. (In truth, I've heard psychologists use the term "tween," but almost always in referring to a much narrower age range, such as ten- to twelve-year-olds. The fact that some are using the term conversationally in any way, though, indicates how some professionals may have been hoodwinked, too.) In reality, no competent professional would dream of lumping children in this age range into the same cohort, as if to infer that eight-year-olds and fourteen-year-olds have something—*anything*—in common developmentally.

Indeed, it was a succession of brilliant twentieth-century psychiatrists and psychologists who revealed that just the opposite was the case. By meticulously carving out the multiple and distinct stages of child and adolescent development—newborn, infancy, toddler, early childhood, middle childhood, late childhood, preadolescence, early adolescence, middle adolescence, and late adolescence—these remarkable men and women wholly "invented" the concept of human *development,* as distinguished from the concept of human *growth.* Whereas growth is merely quantitative, they taught us, developmental changes are qualitative. Children's capacities don't merely expand at each unique age and stage: they are transformed.

Their genius imparted an incalculable gift to families, educators, doctors and other professionals, and most important, children and adolescents of all ages. Before this trailblazing work, it was common to think of children essentially as smaller versions of adults who were simply shorter and knew less. In fact, a popular belief in the 1800s held that inside each sperm cell was a greatly miniaturized human being, just sitting around waiting to find the right uterus to grow in. As the field of child and adolescent development emerged as its own discipline, it became powerfully clear that healthy development at each singular stage relied on successfully completing the previous one, and on quality nurturing by adults who understood and attended to children's unique needs at each and every age and stage. (Only time will tell us the long-term effects on kids who are hurried socially and emotionally right from middle childhood to middle adolescence.) One very concrete and far-reaching result of this work was the establishment of child labor laws, as well as a separate justice system for juvenile offenders, both in recognition of the fact that children are qualitatively different from adults.

The era of the "developing child" also ushered in the era of the "self-aware" and developmentally attuned parent. Today many of us can't seem to get enough education, or read enough books, or go to enough lectures about who our children are and what they need from us. And that's a very good thing. But in addition, we need to be equally as smart and self-aware about the cultural forces conspiring—and that's not too strong a word—against us.

Consider this: identifying the stages of human development took the better part of a century. Decades of research—by such extraordinary luminaries as G. Stanley Hall, Sigmund Freud, Anna Freud, Alfred Adler, Arnold Gesell, Jean Piaget, Erik Erikson, Karen Horney, Harry Stack Sullivan, Abraham Maslow, and the like—were required to piece them together in all their complexity. In my estimation, there is no greater testament to the awesome marriage of marketing and mass media than the extent to which advertisers and merchandisers managed to conflate and collapse them, in a very short fifteen years.

Why Eight- to Fourteen-Year-Olds?

In all fairness, *Newsweek* did acknowledge in 1999 that indeed marketers had played a role in defining "tween identity," by creating products especially for the age group. But it missed the most salient point of all: there had been no such thing as a "tween identity" until marketers made it up.

For sure, marketers' interest was demographic, not developmental. By 1999, eight- to fourteen-year-old kids had reached the 27 million mark, the highest number in two decades. With billions of dollars in their pockets (compared to 1991, a 75 percent increase in spending power for ten-year-olds alone), these impressionable youngsters were easily identified by the industry as an economic powerhouse just waiting to be cultivated. Once someone dreamed up the catchy and memorable moniker "tweens" to capture the message—that eight-year-olds are really just short fourteen-year-olds, with one foot in childhood and the other in full-blown adolescence—the rest was history. A brand-new marketing niche was born, fueled by what turned out to be a wildly prophetic and profitable caveat: "Name them and they will buy," or their parents will buy for them.[6]

But why the emphasis on selling such adult-oriented products to these youngsters? If kids ages eight to fourteen have so much cash on hand, why not simply market-study each age group separately, find out what those particular kids especially like, and go after that? It's all about the math: These kids are only going to be eight to fourteen for a mere seven years; they're going to be adults, well, forever. This wasn't really about "tweens" at all—it was about owning them as market share for the rest of their lives.

Advertisers are hawking way more than "stuff" to kids; they are selling a predetermined worldview of what it looks like to be a happy, successful teen/adult directly to kids just old enough to be able to think that far into the future. And, of course, the stuff marketers are hawking—along with a company's name and logo—is being offered up as the ticket to that very same worldview of success.

Keep in mind, too, that while marketers are busy pushing kids to grow up as fast as they can—and to see themselves as already ready for grown-up products and experiences—experts in the field of child and adolescent health tell us in study after study that what serves kids best is precisely the opposite: postponement. The longer adults can support children in delaying behaviors—including sexual behaviors—that carry potentially serious risks to physical and emotional health, the more likely they are to manage those risks in safe and healthy ways. Every year, even every half year, the research tells us, counts.

A "Done Deed" from the Beginning

The lumping and branding of eight- to fourteen-year-olds as "tweens" was a fait accompli from the start. In the 1999 *Newsweek* article the word appeared matter-of-factly no fewer than thirty times, not once surrounded by quotes. (Ever since, I've been making a total nuisance of myself—sorry, everyone— by badgering people to make those funny finger quotes in the air whenever they say the word out loud.) Descriptions of "tweens" in current publications continue to make these grand generalizations—"tweens are today's teens," "tweens are trying to fit in and at the same time establish their identity," "tweens are seeing themselves as separate from their families"—with no hint whatsoever about whether they refer to the eight-year-old end of the spectrum, the fourteen-year-old end, or somewhere in between. No matter, I guess, since those "tweens" are all the same anyway.

Even websites that publish scary articles about the commercial exploitation of children—including the American Psychological Association and the Campaign for a Commercial-Free Childhood—don't seem to get it. They, too, refer to "tweens" sans quotes around the word, or acknowledgment that it's a marketing handle. A mother who blogs about children and teens, and worries about her kids growing up too fast, wrote recently, "Tweens today are far more 'grown up' than when I was a tween." This I think is what worries me most. Hardly anyone seems to be raising hard questions about the legitimacy of the very concept of "tweens," or even stepping back far enough to notice there might be something *to* question.

My heart really sank in April 2007, when I caught a glimpse of a local parenting magazine on a display rack outside the room where I was about to give a talk. "Tweens and Teens" was its name, and I said to myself, *They've won.*

Even the parenting educators have been taken in. A couple years later I was invited to speak at a booksellers conference "to provide insight into 'tween' readers." As you might suspect, my talk wasn't entirely what the planners were expecting. It took only a few short minutes for them and the audience to "get it," though, as soon as they reminded themselves that eight-year-olds are eight-year-olds, nine-year-olds are nine-year-olds, eleven-year-olds are eleven-year-olds, and none of them are "tweens."

At least my spell checker still gets it, I just noticed, each and every time.

Will the Real Adults Please Stand Up?

One of the pictures on my desk at home is an extended-family photo taken in the late 1800s. Even the youngest children are wearing pretty much the same types of clothing as the grown-ups. It's there to remind me that the "developing child" is a recently identified life form and that, if certain marketers have their way, it may be headed for the endangered species list.

I first set out the photo when I began to notice advertisements for "children's" clothing that mimicked almost exactly the ads on the page opposite for adults. But I started to really worry when adult stores like The Gap began opening junior and then infant/toddler versions of themselves.

This very hour, I went online to see how you might spend a morning shopping conveniently from home at babygap.com. Here's a heads-up: once there, you may actually think you've mistakenly arrived at gap.com instead, since you'll be looking at the very same departments to guide your purchases as the ones listed on adult clothing sites: tops, shirts, sweaters, pants, denim, shoes, socks, outerwear, sleepwear, swimwear, active wear, accessories, etc. I had no idea babies were that discerning! Ironically, some of these hip new outfits for children would be really old hat for generations gone by. Today at babygap.com you can purchase a miniaturized "woven fedora" for your newborn my grandfather might have killed for, and my grandmother would have just *loved* those ruffled bloomer shorts I discovered. For myself, I spotted a very stylish duo of loop-strap sandals in Bali Red and Metallic Gold. (Okay, okay. I admit it. It took everything in me not to copy, paste, and search for a pair in size 6½ medium. In both shades, but of course.)

When a national department store chain first came to my hometown some years ago, one of the flyers that came to our door cleverly divided its youngest customers into three age/marketing groups: teens, tweens, and tee-nies. Be sure to take note of the root word, "teens," in case you haven't realized that your adorable infant or toddler or preschooler or first or second grader is really a "tween" (read: short teen) in training.

Pictures are worth a thousand words, and advertising images, of course, are every bit as powerful as the copy. In one ad I spotted, a little girl is stand-ing several yards in front of a playground, wearing a pink spaghetti-strap belly shirt and short shorts and holding what looks like a cell phone to her ear. It was her facial expression and her "Aren't I sooo cool?" pose that really caught my eye; at first glance, you might have thought she was a miniature teenager, or even her mom, gabbing the afternoon away or spreading the latest gossip with her very best friend.

Lack of Journalistic Step-Back

What alarms me, too, are the matter-of-fact references to "tweens" in re-spected newspapers and magazines. Step-back: Isn't that exactly what we count on these kinds of publications for? One particularly troubling story published in January 2010 was titled "Masculinity in a Spray Can,"[7] about the pressure on younger boys today to groom themselves like much older teens. Ten- to fourteen-year-old boys (and some as young as seven), according to the article, "live in a turbulent, vulnerable world," and are embracing a slew of newly marketed "tween grooming products"—colognes, shampoos, de-odorants, body washes, face washes, body spray, body hydrator, exfoliating washes, gels, and the like—to boost their self-confidence and make them more competitive with girls.

My goodness, all that washing and spraying and hydrating! (Now that's a measure of profound cultural change right there; cleanliness, let alone "irre-sistibility," was definitely not an obsession for my boys at ten.) Though the article is sprinkled with quotes from concerned experts about the jacked-up anxiety marketers are helping to create for younger and younger boys, it's made clear more than once who the real culprits are: "those texting, titillat-ing, brand-savvy female peers, who are hitting puberty even earlier." These girls, the article goes on to say, "are being sexualized at earlier ages, applying lip gloss and wearing racier clothes. Boys, a bewildered developmental step or three behind, are feeling additional pressure to catch up."

And how natural and logical is that? Of course they're desperate to catch up. They're "tweens"—right? Those eight- to fourteen-year-olds in such a "fearsome hurry to grow up"? Axe (makers of Instinct), Old Spice (Swagger), and Dial (Magnetic Attraction Enhancing Body Wash) are just trying to help these poor little guys out of a jam.

But then again, why are those younger and younger girls buying all that lip gloss and all those racy clothes that put these guys in such need of exfoliating wash in the first place? What a racket: a "generation" created wholly out of self-fulfilling prophecies feeding on themselves.

Hey, but What About the Parents?

Right about now—or maybe several pages ago—you've got to be saying to yourself, "Now, wait just a minute. Where in this picture do we place the responsibility of parents?" After all, some adult has willingly been paying for all this "tween"-inspired stuff.

That is *the* question, isn't it?

I'm the first one in line to hold adults, including myself, to our sacred responsibilities in regard to the children in our care. That said, in recent years I've developed a new sense of deep empathy and concern for parents today: *no other generations of parents in history have faced the deliberate and ubiquitous intrusion of multibillion-dollar industries into the privacy of family life and parental authority.*

Moreover, the invention of the "tween" was actually the second wave of the marketing tsunami that has washed over the American families in the past quarter century. The original targets, in fact, were much younger children, and "softening up" their parents—who held the purse strings—was an essential part of that strategy, too.

It's almost impossible to remember a time when practically the only products directly marketed to children were toys and breakfast cereals, and the only venues Saturday morning cartoon shows and big-box stores like Toys R Us. All of that changed in the mid-1980s, shortly after US economists first began looking at trends in corporate income generated *exclusively* by children and preadolescents. Their findings were astounding: whereas in the 1960s two- to fourteen-year-olds directly influenced only about $5 billion a year in parental expenditures, that figure quadrupled to $20 billion by the mid-1970s, and climbed tenfold to $50 billion by 1984.

The child market is an automatic triple play, and if you factor in the power of peer influence, it's a veritable home run. It offers three potentially huge sources of market share: the money in children's pockets, the money in their parents' pockets, and ongoing streams of money for future purchases by both. In what became the fastest expanding market in the country—and eventually globally—for years, retailers and advertisers began blitzing younger and younger children with all manner of products, and all manner of strategies for wearing down their parents' resolve (to solidify the all-important "nag" factor).[8] By 1997, children under twelve were spending a whopping $24 billion of their own money a year, and wielding direct influence over an additional $188 billion of their parents' expenditures. Though I wasn't aware of these figures then, I distinctly remember sensing at the time that the status of American children—as if abruptly altered on a social networking page—had somehow been switched to "consumer," and the role of parents, to "enabler."

I saw one of these classic "nag ads" just the other night: School is just letting out and a frustrated father, standing by his older and decidedly uncool car, is motioning and calling to his son to come over and get in. The son, looking mortified, is seen peeking out from behind a pillar, refusing to budge. Out bounces a cherubic and ecstatically happy-looking eight- or nine-year-old, who practically leaps with joy into his mom's expensive brand-new model, pronouncing that this car is way cool—and so is his mom (unlike the other boy's "loser" of a father, of course) for being smart enough to buy it for him. If kids can have so much sway over really big-ticket items, such as cars, teaching them to manipulate parental purchases of clothes, shoes, gadgets, games, fast food, drinks, sweets, videos, CDs, sporting equipment, cell phones, iPods, and computer-based products is, well, child's play.

Profound Effects on Parenting, Too

Several years ago I participated in a panel presentation for parents at a K–6 school on communicating with children about values. A mother raised her hand during the discussion period to express her exasperation. There was an enormous amount of pressure on her son from peers to buy and experience things, things she knew he either didn't need or was not ready for. Sounding helpless, she was clearly overwhelmed and distraught by this onslaught, both on her son and ultimately on her as a parent. There were plenty of nods around the room.

One of the panelists asked if she could give an example. "Well," she said, "my son is relatively small for his age, and all of his [six-year-old] friends are already out of their booster seats. Here lately, he's been begging and pleading with me to let him ride in the car without it—'only for a block, Mommy, please, please'—so he'll be able to tell his friends 'I did it!' Do you think that would be okay?"

What happened next set off alarms for the panelists. Many in the audience looked stunned by the question, while others—many younger-looking, it seemed—continued to nod knowingly. *Oh no*, I thought to myself. *What's wrong with this picture?* How did we get to the point where some young parents are so beleaguered they don't grasp that adults should never feel pressured or obligated to negotiate over safety with a six-year-old? How did some parents in the room not know this, and how did others (including the many teachers of young children in the room) know it so instinctively?

The experience reminded me of my students who first spoke of a mini–generation gap between them and their younger siblings. I knew then just how successful marketers had been at boosting children's sense of power in the family unit and at undermining their parents' sense of confidence and authority.

Taking Back Our Confidence, and Power

I do think there is a piece of the '60s at play in all this. At its core, the decade was about challenging authority, authority figures, and "the establishment." Much of the country's unrest was fueled by the sentiment that power had been in the hands of a privileged few for too long. The popularized slogan "Don't trust anyone over thirty" became emblematic of many young people's growing suspicion of entrenched, hierarchy-based sources of power, and their embrace of a more truly democratic American ideal.

As a result, we are a much more informal and less traditional society, and family structures have changed gradually along with everything else. Children are very much seen and heard in nearly every aspect of family life, and what they say counts in shaping all kinds of family decisions in ways previously unimaginable. More and more families see themselves as members of a closely knit unit, and less as "adults" and "children" living under the same roof with distinct roles and identities. As a result, in good and not-so-good ways, family dynamics—including family power dynamics—have shifted profoundly. (Marketers know this, too, of course, and use this realignment to inject themselves into family spending patterns.)

As I wrote in Chapter 1, one thing is certain: the more some things change, the more children and adolescents need other things to stay exactly the same. Number one is our certainty about who are the adults and who are the kids, and that they're not the same and definitely not equal.⁹

That certainty is the way parents keep the world right side up for their kids, no matter the outside influences.

The following chapters are intended to help you find—and keep—just that kind of certainty. For now, here are some practical suggestions for dealing directly with outside influences that work against it.

A final word of encouragement: It's very helpful to start raising awareness and setting limits around purchasing and other habits when your kids are young, but having these conversations at any age is useful and important. If you have older kids, who may resist changes in your philosophy, remember—and let them know, too—that as a parent you're always entitled to change course in their (and your family's) best interest.

Things to do:

1. Install a virtual bug zapper of your own that's hypersensitive to the word "tween."
2. Notice whenever children are portrayed in media as consumers, not children. Notice how they look and/or sound and what the emotions on their faces or in their voices convey to children watching.
3. Look out for ads that teach kids how to manipulate their parents into buying them "stuff"; if you have younger children, bring these ads to your kids' attention starting when they are six or seven, if not

younger. Also point out ads that encourage younger siblings to lobby for products that an older sibling owns. Eventually, ask your children to spot these kinds of ads on their own and show them to you. Explain that you're onto these tricks and that they make you mad—how dare advertisers try to get in the middle of children and their parents!—and that you're in charge of the purchases in this family, not outsiders.

4. Talk to your kids early and often about the difference between being a child and being an adult. Explain how growing up works, and how it's going to work in your family, and that deciding on what kids are ready for or not is up to the grown-ups. Make sure they understand that being a certain age doesn't automatically mean you're ready for certain activities and experiences.

5. Look for opportunities to explain that new is not always better, and that in life less is often more. As often as possible, remind children what's really important in life; notice and point out the times your children are happy, content, and having fun when commercial products are not the focus of their attention. Remind them that material things we want and don't or can't have can make us feel very unhappy, but that having them won't necessarily make us feel happy.

6. Explain the word "tween" to your kids. They don't like to be manipulated.

7. Explain the word "entitlement" to your kids as soon as they can understand the concept. Point out that children are absolutely entitled to love and being cared for and to a good education, but not toys, games, electronics, "cool" clothing, and all the other stuff that marketers constantly want to sell them. Make sure they also understand the difference between "needs" and "wants."

8. Visit your children's favorite websites with them. Make a game out of counting all the advertisements you see. Notice when ads pop up from previous sites they've visited and explain how companies share and keep records of where you go online.

9. Practice saying no and sounding as if you *really* mean it. The tone of voice you'll want is a very firm statement of fact—that *you're* in charge—but not filled with emotion (angry, exasperated, etc.). When

children sense emotion in your voice, they know instinctively there might be room for manipulation.

10. When you go into a store where children might find things to buy, make clear the rules about purchases before you enter. Come prepared to leave the store immediately if your kids get whiny and insistent, even if you're not finished shopping. (After a couple times, they'll know you mean what you say about whining being unacceptable.) Or if they're old enough, just walk away and go to another department.

11. Whenever a purchase or activity just doesn't "feel right," especially if you're feeling pressured, go with your gut.

12. Get support from the parents of your children's friends; talk openly with one another and try to reach consensus about what purchases and activities you think are age appropriate, and not. Vow to have one another's backs.

13. Consider seeking professional guidance if you have a particularly hard time saying no and/or sticking to it. You and your children deserve it.

14. Model the values you want your children to value. Notice your own purchasing habits and what they may be communicating to your kids about what you think is important in life.

15. Remember, it's not about the "stuff." It's about being the parent, and holding on tight to your legitimate influence and power.

3

Parenting Is
a Five-Piece Suit

P arents I work with are hungry for advice on what to say to their kids
and how to approach situations that arise in their families around sexuality. Though advice can be very useful, it's not particularly empowering. It doesn't necessarily help you know what to say or do in the next
situation that comes up, when there's likely no one around to ask.

As the English proverb counsels, "Give a man a fish and you feed him for
a day; teach him to fish, and you feed him for a lifetime." This chapter is indeed about teaching you to fish, that is, offering a way of seeing and thinking
about your children—a lens, so to speak—that will help you *advise yourself*
about what to say or do. (First, you have to be willing to touch the fish, which
was the purpose of Chapter 1.) Moreover, it's a lens so wide it can be immediately useful in any and all parenting situations, with virtually any age child,
and whether the issue is sexuality or any other. I know. It sounds too good
to be true.

More than a quarter century ago, I experienced an epiphany that literally transformed my thinking, my work, and my own parenting forever. It handed me a brand-new and concise way of thinking about who children are and what they need most from adults, as well as a means to assess how good a job we're doing. Moreover, it provided a fresh way to understand and explain just why US culture today is so toxic for children and teens and strengthened my resolve to help make change. It was a gift.

What I "got" in that flash was a fundamental distinction between children and adults—in a very particular way—and the answers to these questions: What makes a child a child, and an adult an adult? What specifically about adults enables them to make their way independently in the world, and children not? Who, exactly, are teenagers, and how are they different from "real" adults?

The Need to Be Nurtured

Infants come into the world as totally helpless creatures, except for the awesome ability to communicate their needs very effectively: *Feed me! Change me! Hold me! My stomach is KILLING me! I need to go lie down NOW!* Their basic needs—immediate, concrete, and insistent—are hard to miss. But they also come out of the womb on day one with a much less visible and audible need that goes way beyond mere survival—the need to be well nurtured.

I think of nurturing as synonymous with parenting: To me, "to parent" *is* "to nurture." Nurturing is what enables our children to grow up and away from us and to find their place out in the world as independent adults. (That's why parenting is the only job I can think of where, as soon as you finally succeed, you automatically get fired.) Moving children successfully along from the point of near total dependence *on us* to near total independence *from us* depends in large measure on how well we identify and meet their invisible but ever-present needs for very specific kinds of nurturing.

What a daunting task. Often I meet mothers and fathers who are so overwhelmed by the everyday challenges and stresses of parenting that they sometimes feel paralyzed and out of control. Take a breath, I tell them, and allow me to scale things down to size: the simple truth is that your children—

no matter the age, the situation, or the problem—need at most *only five things* from you at any given moment, on any given day, or, for that matter, in any given year of their childhood or adolescence. Isn't that immediately reassuring to you, too?

Here's the insight I gained years ago. I saw in an instant that what makes a child a child, and not something more, is her or his requirement for nurturing around five universal needs, entirely separate from but every bit as important as basic survival needs. When children first come into the world, I realized, they lack the developmental capacity to meet any of these five on their own, and that's why they need adult nurturers, not simply caretakers. Over many years, as adults nurture children around these core needs, the children gradually learn how to manage each of them independently, and eventually, when they develop the capacity to meet all five wholly on their own, they become adults in their own right. Just as nurturing around these five needs defines us as parents, developing these five capacities will eventually define our children as adults.

I also understood the following corollary: If children have only five fundamental needs, then parents—and teachers and other primary nurturers—have only five fundamental jobs. (Parenting made simple, though not necessarily easy.) Virtually every interaction between adult nurturers and their children can be understood through the prism of these five needs and their corresponding adult roles. Regardless of whether we recognize it, what responsible and responsive grown-ups constantly provide in children's lives are the following: affirmation, information, clarity about values, limits and boundaries, and guidance. That is what we do when we nurture.

Just the other evening I watched a young mother traveling home with her son (two and a half, she told me) on a commuter train from work and preschool. Effortlessly, and with no conscious awareness, she was nurturing up a storm on their long ride home. "You can only have two apricots," she cautioned, "and they're really big so you have to take little bites" (limits). "Great," she said, her eyes full of delight. "You remembered the name of the stop after Farragut North" (affirmation). "Let's see how many more stations you can learn" (information). "What did you like best about school today?" she asked (values). "Be careful getting down off the bench. It's really high" (guidance). And so it went, on and on like this, nonstop, for miles.

These roles are not something adults have to learn. We engage in them naturally and unconsciously if we're at all tuned in to children and their needs, and especially so if we ourselves were well nurtured. By naming them and making them more conscious, we can even more readily interpret our children's needs, and become ever more intentional in how we respond. My best advice to parents is to think of these five roles very deliberately as their walking papers, as a parental job description, if you will, like the one you wished they'd handed you on the way out of the delivery suite.

Whenever they are "on the job," I suggest parents actually visualize themselves wearing these roles as they might a five-piece suit they put on first thing in the morning before they even greet their children for the day. It helps keeps them straight during a time of so much cultural change, pressure, and confusion. It reminds them, and their children, who are the adults in the family and who are the kids. And when it comes to subjects such as sexuality that seem trickier or more challenging than others, it helps them get back their cool and their common sense.

In many respects, most American children are thriving. I can guarantee you that where they are thriving, they are being well nurtured by a caring adult (or that they are incredibly resourceful and resilient by nature). In most ways, however, America's young people are not thriving when it comes to issues of sex, intimacy, and gender; in fact, in those aspects of development many of them are seriously, even dangerously, at risk. Absent consistent and developmentally attuned parenting and age-appropriate schooling, many lack the affirmation, information, clear values, limits, and guidance they need to manage and enjoy their emerging sexuality in healthy ways.

Here's my experience over the past many years: when parents come to understand that the five needs in raising sexually healthy children are the exact same needs involved in raising healthy children, period, they are better able to discover, embrace, and apply their roles around sexuality as well.

Wearing "The Suit": Three Quick Examples

So you pick up your eight-year-old son, Levi after school, feed him a quick sandwich in the car, and drive thirty minutes to drop him off at an afternoon activity. On the way, you comfort him about a mean thing someone said to his friend Jaime at the lunch table (affirmation), tell him you are proud he is such a caring friend (values), help him with his math homework (information), remind him that you'll pick him up at 5 P.M. sharp (limits), and walk him through why he showed up at 5:15 last time, how that made you late for work, and how he's going to keep it from happening this time (guidance). He hops out of the car at your destination, you head off to run an errand, and neither of you is aware of how well he has just been nurtured.

Your daughter Amy is barely twelve. She wants to go to the mall with three or four friends and without any adults. You acknowledge that sounds like fun (affirmation) but that the mall is too big and too crowded a place for her and her friends to just go wandering, especially with no watchful adult eyes (information). Your remind her that safety is always your first concern (values), suggest that she and her friends go to the movie theater at the mall instead, and tell her you'll meet her for ice cream at the store near the movies, not the one at the other end of the mall, ten minutes after the movie lets out (limits). She likes the idea and in fact seems a little relieved but doesn't think her friends will agree. You coach her (guidance) on how to make it sound appealing.

Your son Tony is fifteen. You find a package of condoms in the pocket of a jacket he has asked you, please, to drop off at the cleaners. You run from his room screaming.

Rewind. Your son Tony is fifteen. You find a package of condoms in the pocket of a jacket he has asked you, please, to drop off at the cleaners. You want to run from his room screaming but remind yourself that you just saw condoms, not a big, hairy bear. You put on your "suit" and try hard to look at the situation from his perspective (affirmation). Though he's mature for his age, and you're glad to know he obviously takes physical protection and responsibility seriously (values), you frankly don't know what he knows about emotional intimacy at his age (information), or whether he understands how easy it is to get yourself too deeply into a relationship when you're inexperienced and/or infatuated (limits). You realize you've got a best-case scenario— since you weren't snooping but doing him a favor—and decide to approach him as you would in any other situation where you felt concerned for his welfare (guidance). You're also not entirely sure how you feel about his being in a situation where he even needs to use a condom, and you know you have to think about that (values, again).

Now that wouldn't be so bad, right? (Well, at least you got my point.)

Teachers Are Nurturers, Too

As a teacher I'm also a nurturer. My days, too, are filled with giving affirmation, providing information, highlighting important values, setting limits, and offering guidance. Some days, just for grins, I keep track of every interaction I have with my students while I'm at school. At the end of the day, when I look at the nature of my contacts with kids through the lens of these core needs, they *always* match up perfectly. You would probably discover that's true of the nurturers in your household, too. Give it a try.

Families and schools are the two primary nurturing institutions in children's lives. Both exist, in fact, solely for that purpose. Children bring their five needs from home to school every day, and back again, which makes us de facto partners in raising children around these needs, regardless of whether we consciously recognize it. And if you think about it, the deafening silence around issues of sexuality in many families and schools—where almost every other issue is handled front and center—is glaring and incongruous, if not an outright abdication or even an issue of neglect.

To reframe a point from Chapter 1, adult silence around sexuality leads young people to conclude that everyday nurturers are not accessible or available for that particular kind of nurturing. (I often pass on invitations to provide "one-shot" programs to students at schools I visit more than five hundred miles from home, for fear they may decide the only grown-ups who will talk to them about this subject live in another part of the country altogether. Who are you supposed to talk to after they leave?) And so, they inevitably go elsewhere—friends, peers, popular culture, marketers, the Internet—for answers. What they don't get is nurturing. I am absolutely convinced all we need do to turn this around is "own" these five roles in relation to sexuality, too. Once we do, I predict, marketers will have to shift their focus to some other vulnerable group instead, because our children won't be vulnerable anymore.

When adults don't own their roles around sexuality, I've noticed, it's almost always because they're focused on *their* needs, not children's. The understandable desire to avoid embarrassment, discomfort, inadequacy, anxiety, or controversy can be powerful and even overwhelming, but it needn't be paramount. If our focus truly is on children, our needs frankly become a "so what?" We can work them out some other time and in some other way than choosing not to see or respond to children's basic needs. The mom in the scenario above might very well have felt every one of these emotions—plus maybe sadness and even anger—upon finding those condoms, but when she remembered it was her son's (core developmental, not sexual) needs that were most at stake, she got clear on how to think and respond on *his* behalf. I wonder constantly whether school personnel who refuse to allow certain topics to be discussed in their buildings (often, by the way, the very subjects young people say they most need and want to talk about) recognize whose needs they are really choosing to meet. I hope it would matter.

Five Needs, Five Jobs, and How They Fit Together

Here's the skinny on the five core needs and your corresponding roles. They'll provide the backstory and subtext for the rest of this book.

Affirmation

Affirmation is need number one because, well, it's need number one. Trust in the world, which starts with faith and confidence in us as representatives of the world, is the foundation on which all of children's other needs rest. Not surprisingly, then, affirmation is the most complex need of the five. It has numerous components, each of equal and singular importance.

Attention

As everyone knows, children are desperate for attention; it's their major source of love, safety, comfort, and acknowledgment. Our attention tells them they exist and that they matter. If it's not forthcoming in positive ways, they'll try anything to get it, and take whatever kind they can get. For a child who feels neglected, the adage "negative attention is better than no attention" is a no-brainer.

Attention for a child is a two-way street, and not getting it is a double whammy: Children are not just needy for attention *from us*; they are compelled intuitively to pay attention *to us*. "Look at me," they say in part, "because I need to look at you!" It's by watching us attend to their needs that they learn—very gradually—to do those things for themselves. In other words, they are hardwired for nurturing.

I read an article recently about parents using smart phones as electronic babysitters because very young children quickly become mesmerized by the constant two-way interactions these devices can create. One of my fears about this technology in children's lives is how intensely it meets their instinctive need for looking and being looked at, for attending and being attended to. To what degree, I worry, might it diminish their intuition or motivation to seek the attention of adult nurturers, who themselves, let's face it, may be continually preoccupied with their own computer and cell phone screens? What's more, let's remember, all too often this gadgetry is programmed by adults who manipulate the seductive power of interactivity for the purpose of selling both products and a global worldview that will invite more and more spending. In truth, no one can even pretend to know the immediate and long-term effects of this grand experiment in child development. But to the extent that that preprogrammed interactions provide a substitute for the intimacy and spontaneity of a nurturing relationship, it can't be good.

On the last day of school, while walking to my car to leave campus, I spotted a former student—himself now a dad—walking toward the building, hand in hand with his four-year-old, to pick up an older sibling. Right away I sensed the two-way connection between them. As David guided his son across the parking lot, he scanned it, pointing out novel things to look at along the way and watching out for oncoming cars. From time to time the boy glanced up at David's face briefly but intently in perfect tandem, I noticed, with the slightest elevation or nuance in his dad's voice.

Two-way nurturing personified. There is no substitute for *that* in a child's life.

Unconditional Acceptance and Love

One of the great insights of modern psychiatry and psychology is the distinction between *acceptance* and *approval.* Unconditional acceptance—to me, the operational definition of love—means taking someone or something as it is, with no need or desire whatsoever to change it. Acceptance is an absolute and qualitative state of being. Just as you can't be a little bit pregnant, you can't be a little bit accepting. Approval and disapproval, on the other hand, exist along a qualitative scale. They rest on judgment—relative to a particular point of view—about how someone or something should be. The realization that parental acceptance *and* parental disapproval can coexist at any moment can be transformative. Recognizing that you can experience total acceptance *toward your child* while also feeling totally disapproving *of his behavior* can take a lot of the angst (and guilt) out of disciplining children and teens. It also means you're clear on the difference between need number one (affirmation) and needs three (values) and four (limits).

Many parents who are clear on the difference between acceptance and approval take extra care to "criticize the conduct, not the child." They remind themselves to communicate, "bad behavior!" not "bad girl!" or "bad boy!" (even though declaring the latter might feel ever so much more satisfying at the moment). They're also careful to "praise the behavior, not the child," since they know that saying "good girl" gives the clear message that a child could just as easily be a "bad girl."

Once I was discussing this point with a group of parents when a mother raised her hand and asked (in an ever-escalating tone of voice, and only half in jest), "Do *you* mean to tell *me* that I have to feel *accepting* toward my fifteen-year-old son, who, I just found out, went and charged $200 worth of pornography on my credit card and then *lied* to me about it?" At this point someone turned to her and said softly, "Well, yes." "I was afraid you were going to say that," the woman said with an audible sigh and a (half) smile. She knew she still loved and accepted her son absolutely, and was obliged in fact to do so (hence, the sigh)—even when she absolutely deplored his behavior.

Some of you may recall when grown-ups were not at all careful with you and caused you to feel as if *you* were the problem—*you* were bad—not your behavior. The pain of those experiences may linger, or throb, even today. Children need to feel adults' love and total acceptance for who they are at all times, even when their behavior is deplorable. It's their birthright.

All parents remember the first time they looked deeply into their new-born's eyes—or the eyes of a baby or child they brought into their home—and fell in love. Who we fall in love with is that brand-new, precious, perfect, complete, and utterly unique in the history and future of the world human being, who just *is*. (And who is still in there, even when his behavior is rude, inconsiderate, irresponsible, selfish, deceitful, or otherwise obnoxious.) That's the part of children we owe our undying, unconditional acceptance.

But their behavior? That's another matter altogether. For that, approval and/or disapproval from caring adults, as needed, is essential.

Validation

Validation is so simple we can easily miss its significance, especially for children. To validate someone is to send the message, "I 'get' you. I see who you are. You exist." It's about holding up a mirror to another person's life and reflecting it back, without distortion or judgment. Active listening,[1] which entails both focusing on emotion in another person's communication and reflecting it back to her in your own words, is a powerful form of validation. So is making a point to ask questions about the images and colors in a child's drawing, rather than saying, "What a pretty picture!" For very young children, who totally lack the cognitive ability to step outside their own heads and look back at themselves, our validation is how they initially come to know and accept themselves; for older kids, it's also a way of helping them know who they are becoming.

Validation, like acceptance, has nothing to do with approval or disapproval; it's merely an acknowledgment of *what is*. When offered with genuine interest, it meets people's need to be noticed, valued, known, and accepted, and it almost always feels good. It's a powerful way to engender trust and open up honest and real communication with everyone, including children and teenagers. I frequently walk into classrooms full of kids I've never met before to talk with them about really sensitive and personal issues. I learned a long time ago that if I just sit back and listen for a bit and then simply reflect back or ask questions about a few of the things I happened to notice while waiting for class to start, we're already off to a good start. It's quite miraculous, really, the power of simply getting what *is*.

Taking Perspective

Perspective-taking is what underpins the ability to empathize. Whereas sympathy involves feeling *for* someone, empathy is the ability to feel *with* someone. To empathize with someone else's life, to feel what *she or he* feels, we first have to "suspend" ourselves—put "us" on the back burner, so to speak—long enough to experience the world through *her or his* eyes.

Taking on a child's or adolescent's perspective can be especially challenging. First, it's easy to forget that children and teens don't think like we do, which is to say, they don't have the brain capacity to process information in the same way as adults, so they often draw vastly different conclusions than we would in the exact same situation. (Their relatively limited life experience plays a role here, too.) Second, we can't "see" children's brain development, so we tend to take our cues more often from those aspects of development—physical, social, emotional—we *can* see, even though the way children and adolescents think and reason is often the ticket to understanding how they see the world. (Just because a girl is relatively tall, for example, doesn't mean she's particularly mature in any other way; we don't want to expect too little of our kids, but we need to be cautious about overestimating their abilities, too.) Finally, we aren't necessarily the most objective "readers" of what's in our children's minds; the emotional staples of any parent's life—love, fear, anger, and guilt—can easily lead to misinterpretation, faulty projections, or even denial of our children's own reality.

What's more, children and teens—no matter how hard we try to see their point of view—don't always want us to know. They may deliberately hide or misrepresent what they're really thinking. And then go figure.

Sexuality is a topic where adults are especially prone to project, out of their own anxiety or discomfort, what they *think* children are thinking (or what they're doing, or about to do). The old joke comes to mind about the young child who asks where she came from (the answer she was looking for was "Chicago") but the parent, sweating bullets, gives a lecture on the birds and the bees and bunny rabbits, and eventually humans, complete with diagrams and a video. My favorite real-life example is my cousin's ten-year-old daughter, who asked if she was going to "get hair" (you can guess how far my over-anxious cousin, looking for an "in" to talk about puberty, went with that one) when the girl was actually worried about getting hair in her nose like Great-Uncle Lou.

Though these kinds of stories are funny and make us laugh, mostly at ourselves, projecting our own "stuff" onto the questions children and adolescents commonly ask sometimes has the effect of shutting down communication altogether. When a teen asks a simple question out of curiosity about a topic such as birth control, for instance, but a parent reacts out of his or her own anxieties—"Just *why* do you want to know about *that*?!"—it may just be, very sadly, the last question that teen brings up *ever*. Reminding ourselves to put "us" on the back burner (otherwise known as the parental art of tongue-biting) until we've taken a look through our children's eyes on the world is always—and I rarely say always—the right thing to do. In this example, a direct answer to the question, in a matter-of-fact tone of voice, is all the teen is looking for, and also what will keep her or him, I promise, coming back for more.

Developmental "Knowing"

Most parents work hard at knowing their children as individuals better than anyone else in the world, and that's a good thing. There's another kind of "knowing" that's just as important—knowing and affirming your growing child as someone who is passing through a particular and unique *developmental stage*. Let's say your daughter is turning eight today. Knowing as much as you can about her distinctive physical, social, emotional, and intellectual characteristics as *an* eight-year-old, not just *your* eight-year-old, helps you nurture her in all the ways that will support her next year in becoming the sturdiest and most capable nine-year-old she can possibly be. (That's what building a school's curriculum is about, too.)

In potent ways, as we've seen, American culture does not affirm who children are developmentally; that's why Chapter 2 is so important as a backdrop for the rest of this book. Knowing exactly who your children are developmentally helps them, and it also helps you become an effective "counter-culture" nurturer. "Developmental knowing" is the subject of Chapter 4, coming up next.

Information

All grown-ups understand the responsibility of adults to pass on to children the wisdom of the ages. Even at the dizzying pace that information and technology literally explode around us (I knew I was a dinosaur more than twenty-five years ago, when our four-year-old said "Just push *that*, Mommy!" as I labored over our cute little Apple IIE), we're still their primary source of knowledge and insight about how life works in the real world. No computer, or "virtual world," can teach that.

We are also our children's first and most important educators. In their earliest years we give them volumes and volumes of information both incidentally—in the process of life itself—and deliberately, as we increasingly make a point of teaching them new things every single day. And well before they ever take their first steps into a school building, we also teach them how to learn practically everything else. (Take a bow.) We do this effortlessly, and for the most part unconsciously, because that's what nurturers naturally do.

We also get very good at knowing how to explain things on just the right level a particular child or adolescent can understand, because we get so much practice at it. And if we don't quite get it right the first time, we often can use our intuition and good common sense to come up with a do-over that will better hit the mark. And think about the huge range of topics we eventually address with our kids from age zero to eighteen. (I've yet to meet a teacher who has taught all those topics and ages.) Truthfully, *all* parents deserve a teaching certificate (and a bonus) by the time their children graduate from high school.

Clarity About Values

To babies and toddlers, everything is possible, and everything is equal. That, by the way, is a major cause of temper tantrums: What do you mean I can't have *that*, or try *this*? Don't you people know *everything* is possible?

It's only by experiencing and trying out new things that young children begin to discover—Oh, I get it!—that everything is *not* equal: Some things I like and some things I don't. Some things taste or feel really good, but not everything. Some things I do make my dads look happy with me, and some things make them look mad. Some things are okay to put in my mouth, and some things will make me sick or choke.

Recognizing that not everything is equal is how children learn to make value judgments, an essential prerequisite for functioning independently in the world. Life is not neutral. We have to know what is good for us and for our well-being, and what is harmful; what kinds of behaviors will be received favorably by others, and what kinds, rightfully or not, will provoke anger and upset; who we can trust, and who not; what things fit our interests and capacities really well, or not so much; what seems like fun in the short run but might work against our best interests in the future. We also need the know-how to make honorable judgment calls in matters that involve morally right or wrong choices, and the ability to think in terms of abstract values and ethical principles.

Psychologists often describe adolescence as a "second toddlerhood," or as my friend describes it, "the 'terrible twos' on steroids." Though separated in time by ten or more years, both stages are essentially about exploring a larger world on brand-new terms, and learning to make brand-new kinds of value judgments. Only this time around, young people need primarily to look *inward* to discover what is most of value in life. Indeed, teens may need to test out almost everything all over again—check out the last sentence two paragraphs up, in the context of teen drinking or smoking, for example—and not chiefly for the purpose of "testing" adult boundaries, as we often assume: Every new experience conceivably becomes a testing ground for rethinking *themselves.* To come through adolescence, ultimately, as separate individuals with their own unique identity, they need all of these opportunities to reconstitute a set of values and beliefs that match up with who they really are and who they are becoming, not their parents' or even their peers' ideas about who they should be.

For parents trying to make the adjustment to having an adolescent in the house, it's really useful to remember what being a teenager and being a toddler have most in common: every bit as intensely as toddlers are driven to toddle (just imagine trying to hold one tightly in your lap when they really, really want to get down and explore), adolescents are driven to think and make value judgments on their own terms, which doesn't mean, by the way, that they want full autonomy or total control. They still want and need us in their lives, no matter how often they roll eyes or slam doors—but they also need and deserve respect for their very normal and increasing desire for independence.

Being clear and very direct with our children—continuously—about what *we* think and value is just as essential. Again, young children at first see everything in life as equal and neutral; out of all those limitless possibilities, how will they know which relationships, behaviors, activities, rules, places, things, ideas, experiences, beliefs, values, ideals, etc., are most important if we don't tell or show them? Adolescents, too, need (and want!) to know where we stand on the important stuff as well, even if they don't always show it or rarely seem to agree with us. No matter how mature they might be for their age, the world is still a scary and unknown place in ways large and small and they need help scaling it to size—that is, knowing what's most important to pay attention to. Remember as well that adolescents are developmentally obliged to push and pull against parental values, to define and launch their own separate identity. What supports them most is their knowing *exactly* what they're pushing and pulling against, so they have a definable target to work with. Otherwise, trust me, they end up trying to guess at it, to give themselves something to work with. That's a lot murkier and inevitably slows down and complicates the process.

Setting Limits

As I've said probably a thousand times, limits and boundaries are those brackets we put around children's lives to keep them safe and healthy. A baby's crib, for example, is a truly wonderful metaphor for setting limits: the space inside represents the maximum degree of freedom we allow an infant unless we're right there in person to keep watch. The art of parenting going forward, in very large measure, is about *best guessing* how and when to push those boundaries out, just a little bit, or more, and when to hold tight; when to stand by "just in case" and when to let go altogether and watch our children soar.

For me, the image of an excited parent motioning and encouraging a baby's first steps—all the while primed to leap in a flash to the rescue—captures precisely what it means to nurture around limits and boundaries. As the parent of two grown sons, I remember reliving that exact same combination of caution and exhilaration, and on occasion terror or sadness, every time each of them took another "first step" away from us and into a larger world. Last June I saw all of that, and more, on my colleague's face at his son's high school graduation.

The limit-setting role parents play is the most concrete of the five, and the easiest to recognize as a "cradle through adolescence" proposition. The issues around which we establish boundaries for children and adolescents change profoundly across the developmental spectrum, but the basic need for borders, fences, and guardrails is ongoing and ever present.

Setting limits around sexuality in children's lives, and gradually teaching them to internalize their importance, is an ongoing effort, too. When children are very young, for example, the concepts of privacy and personal space are out of their cognitive reach, but when they're five or six, we can readily teach them to knock on closed doors and to keep their clothes on in public spaces, and help them begin to sort out the proper times and places for talking about—or enjoying—their sexual parts. As the years pass, we'll find ourselves setting limits around nudity in the family (my rule of thumb is that sooner or later someone will start to feel uncomfortable and parents or their kids will know that it's time), "sex play" with other kids, language, media consumption, technology use, and what's appropriate for them to wear and play with, and not. As children approach adolescence, we'll be doing some of the same, as well as devising parameters for their expanding social lives, including issues around curfews and supervision of parties and "dates." We'll need to talk about sexual boundaries and limits, too—increasingly so as they mature—and explain what it means to respect other people's sexual boundaries and your own.

Ample research makes clear that even as parents (legitimately) begin to lose direct control over their teenagers' whereabouts and decisions, they can—with deliberate effort—retain considerable *influence on what, and how, their children ultimately decide.* According to many studies, one especially effective way is to conscientiously monitor where your children are, whom they're with, what they're doing, and what kind of adult supervision is present when they're out and about on their own. Monitoring your children's activities in your own home when no adults are present is just as important (and effective) since many kids engage in potentially risky behaviors—including sexual behaviors—under their parents' roofs when work and other commitments keep adults away. Stating your expectations, and then following through by arranging for routine check-in—via phone or video calling—is more powerful than it may seem. It reminds your kids that you're thinking about them and their welfare, and makes your presence felt even when you're a distance away.

The Not-So-Simple Act of Saying No (and Meaning It)

When our kids hear inner confidence when we say no, they are less likely to manipulate us into "Well, okay, yes." We communicate most of our power as parents not by what we say, but how we say it; a tone of voice that broadcasts firmly yet calmly, "I mean what I say and I say what I mean," is the key regardless of the words. My dog, for example, doesn't get words, but he sure gets tone of voice, and I'm still searching for the right one. Comparing animals to people is risky business, but I know a pregnant woman who I'm convinced will make a wonderful limit setter with her kids. I can say no to my dog three different ways and half the time he still does pretty much what he pleases. She says it once, and he stops in his tracks. What he hears in her voice, I'm sure, is there's no point to his usual tricks, not with this one. If I weren't so embarrassed I would ask her to make me a tape.

When parents consistently find it difficult to say no to their kids, the power dynamic in the relationship can shift in ways that invite perpetual conflict and unpleasantness. Kids who know that if they just push harder, or shift tactics, they can pretty much get their way can become relentless in their demands. Children and teens, generally, often don't distinguish clearly between their wants and their needs, but those empowered by unclear boundaries may develop a sense of entitlement to the point that they continuously hold their parents hostage with behavior that says, "I have to have it, or else I'll make things really miserable around here." Understandably, parents may choose the path of least resistance by giving in, only to reinforce the pattern. A helpful outsider, like a counselor or therapist, can help get the balance of power back in check. It's important to remember always that regardless of their behavior, *internally* children and teens really do want us to be the ones ultimately in charge.

Remember, too, that in the process of setting limits, we teach kids how to set them for themselves. Perhaps you know adults who don't get the importance of setting limits and boundaries around their own lives, or even know how to set them; they aren't fully grown up and sadly may never be. If you think about it, making decisions about how much is too much (or too little) and how far is too far (or not far enough) is what capable adults—including parents—do virtually all day every day: Offered a job? How much does it pay? There's a police car behind me—do I need to slow down? I don't think that at fifteen you can process that movie. That's it—I've had enough of his rudeness. I'm going to complain. Ten kids are too many to invite. How about we say eight? That milk is too expensive, but the juice is on sale. I've got *just enough* time to stop by and see her. That car is too close! That skirt is too short! If you're going to be later than ten, let your dad know. That water's too deep, come out of it *right now*! Nah, kissing is okay at your age, but not intimate touching. And so on, and so on, and so on. Keep track for yourself one day—you'll just be amazed.

What? You don't have that kind of time? Okay, half a day.

Anticipatory Guidance

Everybody needs consultants. Tomorrow, since I'll be home from school in the morning, I will call the plumber, the cable company, and my dog's vet. The kitchen sink is leaking, my Internet is in and out, and poor Misha's moping around like he's lost his best friend and not eating a thing. The numbers are right next to the phone on my desk so I can get to them first thing.

Children and adolescents need consultants and guides, too. Their very narrow range of life experience puts them at great disadvantage in finding the right kind of resources and know-how to solve problems and take care of themselves, and that's certainly a key role for adults in their lives. But children also need a totally different kind of guidance, one that adults don't require nearly as much, and that's *anticipatory guidance.*

Even as teenagers, young people have a relatively limited ability to project themselves into the future, think about what *might* happen in certain circumstances, what *might* happen if those things were to happen, what *might* happen if *those* things were to happen, and so on. First of all, the future isn't here yet, and younger minds have difficulty grasping what can't be experienced concretely through the senses. Second, the ability even to think in terms of probability or assign likelihood to future events—something adults do all day every day and just take for granted—requires more higher order thinking than children and many adolescents can muster, especially when they're under stress (or the influence of alcohol or other drugs).

Being able to think ahead in terms of abstract possibilities, or not, is a matter of time and brain development. It's also one of the most basic *qualitative* distinctions between children—including teenagers—and adults. The wise expression, "Parents: The Frontal Lobe," says it all. Children need us to think ahead for them in ways they can't yet do for themselves.

Making the Transition from Limits to Guidance

My earliest recollection of offering my older son anticipatory guidance was the second day I dropped him off at kindergarten. He hopped out of the car (no booster seats back then) and headed toward the entrance. "Wait, come back here a second," I called out. "Tell me again where we put your lunch money, so you don't forget like yesterday." I could have switched to the option of sending in a check for the entire half of the year, but I decided to trust him—with a little bit of help—to do something important on his own.

That's what anticipatory guidance is all about—handing your child over, in small ways and big, to herself or himself. It's a good thing to watch yourself do this, little by little, as your children mature, so you can keep track of what it is you look for in deciding they're ready. Doing so will help you chronicle, for you and for them, their growing sense of ownership and responsibility, and also help you better explain to yourself and to them the yardsticks you use whenever you decide to give them more freedom, or not.

Arriving at the right balance between limits and guidance is an art, not a science, especially when your children are teens. And here of course is the scary part: at the very same age teens begin to crave more and more independence, and to resist limits they think are too strict, they're also more likely to find themselves in situations where risky choices are more easily accessible. Parents who recognize their teens' need for both freedom and limits, and who know how to keep recalibrating the balance as their children mature, make the transition to freedom most successfully and with the least amount of conflict and risk.

All along the way, it's important to walk children through what the future might look like when they get there and have to cope on their own, by helping them identify the things that might or could happen that they may not know to anticipate. Sexual decisions are among the earliest and most important ones young people make by themselves (we're not likely to be there when they do), and they need and deserve clear anticipatory guidance around those possibilities, too. When we help prepare our kids for the variety of situations they're likely to face around sexual choices, fundamentally we're not "talking to them about sex," but fulfilling our role as their chief anticipatory guide, just as we do around everything else.

A Final Note: Preventing Child Sexual Abuse

"Good touch/bad touch" programs for children can help children recognize and verbalize whether physical contact with another person—of any kind—feels okay to them or not. And that's a good thing. In the service of child sexual abuse prevention, though, I think it's a misguided and perhaps even harmful approach. The way to prevent child sexual abuse is through adult behavior, not children's; what's required is vigilance, research, and monitoring, to make certain that children are supervised continuously under the watchful eyes of trusted adults. Most sexual abuse programs focus on giving anticipatory guidance *to children* about what to do if they are ever in an uncomfortable or scary situation, not on helping adults set the kind of limits around children's lives that will keep them safe. I worry that children come away with the idea that *they* are responsible for keeping themselves safe; then if something terrible happens, they may feel they are to blame.

Moreover, in schools where sexual abuse prevention is the only "sex education" young children receive, the tone set for this topic will be one of danger and threat. And since most programs don't specifically name sexual parts (they're referred to usually as "private parts" or "the part of your body covered by a bathing suit"), they instill a sense of secrecy, "otherness," mystery, and perhaps even shame about parts of their body we're encouraging children to be open about in the first place. Finally, the focus of these programs is often on "stranger danger," whereas in reality, the vast majority of child molesters are known to the family in an intimate way, because that's how they win the trust they need to gain private access to the child. The current level of overblown hysteria over "sexual predators" trolling the Internet—or residing in the next zip code over—in search of children and teens to exploit worries me as well. Though Internet stalking is certainly a problem to be aware of, the risks are minuscule compared to the most prevalent dangers for children online, such as cyber bullying.

My own instinct is to include the issue of molestation within a long list of other health and safety messages we deliver to young children all the time in matter-of-fact, in-context ways. Here's an example: "Most adults love children and want to protect them. It's important to know that a very small number of adults do not have children's best interests in their heart. Here's how you can tell if an adult is not treating you correctly, and if that ever happens, tell me right away, even if they tell you not to or make scary threats." Sexual touching then becomes one of many examples you can give.

By the way, people don't have private parts and public parts. They just have parts, and some of those parts *we keep more private* than others most of the time. That's a concept all children can grasp and learn to apply.

Five Needs/Five Roles: Sexuality Is No Different

The five needs/five roles paradigm is the very best way I know to support children's healthy sexual development, and the quickest way to wrap your head around the process. What's more, if ever you are really stumped or stuck or stopped in your tracks by this subject, here's what I hope you remember: even though the situation in front of you may feel, look, and sound like it's about sexuality—for instance, the unforgettable moment when my eight-year-old son asked, "Mom, are you and my father planning on having sexual intercourse anytime soon?"—it isn't. No matter the particular challenge in front of you, or whatever the situation *seems* to be about, it's always really about your children bringing to you one or more of their five generic needs. And from time to time—*oh, by the way*—those needs are going to be related to sexuality.

P.S.: What my son was looking for was not information about anybody's sex life, but reassurance (affirmation) that his parents had no immediate plans to bring another alien into the family, like the little brother who at that very moment was sitting next to him driving him nuts in the backseat of my car. (I realized this after I almost ran the car off the road.)

Here's another piece of advice to help get your common sense back, and put your "suit" back on, in a jiffy: Pretend the situation in front of you is not about sexuality at all, but about some other challenge instead. Then think about what you would do in *that* case. Once, for example, I walked into my bathroom and happened upon my four-year-old son (the other one) playing in the sink. He had filled the basin with water, taken two tampons from the box, removed the cellophane wrappings, tied the two strings together, plopped them into the water, and—voila!—he'd invented a nifty new game of tugboat. (By the way, I always used to leave my tampon box out on the bathroom shelf, for two reasons. One, I thought its presence might lead to some fruitful conversation—it did!—and two, I never saw much point in putting away something you were only going to need again, in what, another twenty-eight days or so.)

But happening upon this particular "teachable" moment, I did something no self-respecting sexuality educator would ever do: I freaked! And to make matters worse, and please don't tell anybody, I then went and said something really, really lame: "Isn't it time for lunch?" Still obsessing over the thing hours later—I just couldn't make sense of my reaction—I decided to take my own advice and pretend it wasn't about tampons at all. I said to myself: Okay. If there were another object in this house that was this small, this nontoxic, this disposable, this biodegradable, this inexpensive, this much fun to play with, and could also teach something interesting and useful about Archimedes' principle and boats, would I hesitate?

I went out the next day and bought him his own box.

How to Wear the "Suit"

If you take a look back at Chapter 2 with the "five-piece suit" metaphor in mind, a plain truth jumps right off the pages: When it comes to sexuality, American society at large provides children and adolescents *the opposite* of what their core needs dictate—distortions about who they are developmentally; misleading and wholly inadequate information; a mess of mixed messages about values; disregard for sexual limits and boundaries; and a near-absence of systematic guidance on how to live a satisfying, caring, healthy, and ethical sexual life. But here's the most important point of all: Very little about "society" really matters, when we—the immediate adults in their lives, to whom they are always looking unless we don't or won't engage—put that suit on every single day.

So, here are some key parts of the job—a skill set or job description, if you will—with detailed guidance to follow in the next five chapters, one for each need. You might want to keep them handy as a checklist while you're getting used to "role-based" versus "sex-based" approaches.

Affirmation

- Paying attention to children's sexual and gender development each day, and at every stage
- Inviting and validating your children's questions, ideas, feelings, and opinions about sexuality
- Putting on hold your reactions and responses to what they say and do long enough to look at the situation through their eyes first
- Understanding your children's true developmental capacities and limitations, and resisting media and other pressures to the contrary

Information

- Knowing *how* children and teens think, and *what* they really want and need to know about sexuality at different ages and stages, and rejecting folk "wisdom" to the contrary
- Providing basic factual information in helpful ways, using direct and accurate language
- Expecting your children to engage with you in thinking deeply about issues of sex, gender, and reproduction, and following through on this often

Clarity About Values

- Distinguishing various ways of thinking about sexual values, and knowing which ones best fit you and your family
- Stating clearly your beliefs, ideas, and values regarding sexuality to your children, and then being prepared to listen nonjudgmentally to their reactions
- Helping your children to clarify their own developing attitudes and values connected to sexuality and to identify the values embedded in media messages to which they're exposed

Setting Limits

- Deciding on and sticking to age-appropriate limits around your children's social (including online) lives, knowing how and when to move them out (or in), and when and how to negotiate (or not)

- Teaching your children why and how sexual limits and boundaries are important, how to decide where to place them, and how to communicate them clearly

Anticipatory Guidance

- Anticipating new experiences your children will move into in the near and more distant future, socially and sexually, and building in the basics they'll need to manage them well
- Educating your children explicitly about the ingredients of a satisfying, caring, healthy, and ethical sexual life

A Case Study: Frank

Frank is a very engaged and proud father of three children, eight, eleven, and barely fifteen. We met when he attended a parenting course I teach. He is one of my heroes.

One early evening, Frank and his oldest child, Elisabeth, were catching up casually after dinner about school, her friends, an upcoming vacation, and other stuff. In the midst of the conversation, she said the following, in the same tone of voice she might have used in announcing, say, an upcoming dental appointment: "Dad, you know, I think pretty soon I'll start going to parties like the ones kids at school go to." (Up to this point, she'd been pretty much a stay-at-home-on-weekends kid.) "And," she continued, "I'm probably going to get drunk there and give guys 'blow jobs,' too."

To say that Frank, who had never before discussed *anything* with Elisabeth about sex (or alcohol), was unprepared for this sudden declaration of independence would be the understatement of the new century. Truly, it rocked him and his world to the core. From his telling, he stood there literally speechless, and motionless. (A full-blown "there's a big, hairy bear in my living room" stress reaction.) How was he supposed to respond? Everything he thought he knew about his life, his child, his ground of being as a parent had just been yanked out from under him, or so it felt. He hated his own helplessness, because he took such pride in being a good father.

When Frank first brought up the story in class, he couched it in very general terms, only later quoting Elisabeth more precisely. He was embarrassed to even utter the phrase "blow job," let alone to admit his daughter had used it and in what context. It seemed a relief, though, to actually say and thereby "own" the words that had made him so crazed, and it prompted another parent to ask, "Frank, why do you think she said that to you?"

The lightbulb over Frank's head switched on almost immediately. It was obvious to everyone. He'd suddenly found the "step-back" he needed to regain his sea legs as a parent, and to reclaim his authority as the adult in the conversation. And he knew exactly what to do: put *Elisabeth*, not "blow jobs," back at the center of the exchange. The sexual implications of her announcement were (practically) beside the point, he realized. This was an "oh, by the way" moment between the two of them; Elisabeth was asking for some serious nurturing, and in this instance, *oh, by the way,* it just happened to be around sexuality.

Later on in class we defined the five needs/five roles concept, and used Frank's experience to try it out. Indeed, why *had* Elisabeth said that to her dad? What was going on in *her* world and in *her* head? After considering several suggestions from the group, Frank reached the conclusion that his daughter probably was feeling really scared (affirmation). Here she was, relatively inexperienced socially, but thinking it was time for her to get with the program, or at least what she thought was the program. She'd probably heard sensationalized and even salacious versions of what "people" do at "parties"—for which she apparently was bracing herself—and needed support (more affirmation) and an honest reality check (information). She'd said something really provocative, maybe because she didn't know how else to bring up the situation, and most likely to provoke a strong reaction so she could size up her dad's opinions (values) and test his willingness to say, "No, I don't think so" (limits and boundaries). Mostly, she was asking for guidance: "Okay, I'm going to take a plunge into some really tricky water here. *Help!*"

Frank did way more than go home and have a "do-over" with Elisabeth. He hung a sign on his "suit," permanently, that says, "The sexuality educator is now in." Each week, in some form or another, he took home all the exercises from class to the dinner table—to his squirming wife, three children, *and* mother-in-law—where he played the role of facilitator, gracefully presiding over some really fascinating discussions. He was fearless, indomitable, and gleeful through it all, and became the class's hero, and inspiration, too. I wish you could see him in action.

By the way, the "do-over" went exceptionally well. He began by being honest that she'd taken him by surprise with her "blow job" comment (he chose to use the language she'd used, to take away its power in the conversation, but added he thought the term was demeaning, and why, and that he would use the term "oral sex" instead). His candor put them both at ease. He asked Elisabeth to tell him what she'd heard about the parties she'd mentioned, and asked how she felt about the stories. The other parents in the class had been right. She was scared but didn't know how else she could become more social, and didn't know how to ask for advice. The stories were likely exaggerated, Frank told her, and added that plenty of kids socialize without doing things they're uncomfortable with. Elisabeth was visibly relieved, and together they came up with other ideas for expanding her circle of friends. Frank was thrilled.

The Power of
Knowing What You Know

The relationship between a nurturer and a child is totally different from any other kind. We might play each of these roles from time to time in other relationships, but they don't define, prescribe, or limit the nature of those relationships. Imagine treating your peers (or your grown children) the way you act toward your kids. Telling your neighbor you won't meet her for coffee until she has done her laundry, or insisting that your grown sister or brother wear something "more appropriate" to the office, just wouldn't fly. And partners or spouses don't rely on us to teach them right from wrong, run them through the paces before every important business meeting, or check homework. (If so, they need a nurturer or mentor, not a partner.) Grown-ups generally are expected to be able to do these things on their own; that's why they're grown-ups.

You've been living these roles since your children came into your life, even if you've never once noticed or named them. (If you're a man reading this book, you may not know you have two seminal vesicles, but they work just fine anyway.) But there's power in this kind of awareness—in knowing what you know. Here are more than a dozen ways you can use the five needs/five roles paradigm to become an ever clearer and more intentional parent.

- As a unifying philosophy/approach to parenting that can work seamlessly throughout your growing child's life
- To keep your immediate focus on kids' needs, rather than on your own
- To avoid being on "auto pilot" as a parent and to take a more proactive approach
- As a reminder to step back in charged situations, so you can choose to respond to your children more deliberately and less reactively
- To assess your "job performance" as a parent and make course corrections
- As a check on how well you're attending to all five needs in equal balance with one another (they are a package deal)
- As a focal point for conversation between co-parents about consistency in approach
- For making a quick "differential diagnosis" to uncover which one or more (sometimes it's all five!) of your child's needs are present, and to decide where best to start
- To avoid confusing one need with another in murky situations
- To create "nurturable" moments, by attending first to whichever need is present, and then moving on to touch base with the other four
- To provide clarity and security for your children about what they can expect from you as their parent and the roles you will "wear"
- To underscore the difference between being your children's parent and being your children's "friend" (friends are equals; parents are nurturers)
- To remove some of the angst in your family life, by "depersonalizing" conflict situations ("I am bound to do these things because I am your parent")
- As a tool for anticipating what children's core needs—and your roles—will look like in the next developmental stage
- As a reminder that the ultimate goal in meeting children's needs is to teach them how to meet them skillfully on their own, so they can eventually fire you

And oh, by the way, everything on this list applies to sexuality, too.

4

Affirmation: Our Children as Sexual Beings

Sexuality educators—myself included—are inclined to say things like, "People are sexual beings from birth on." Americans have great difficulty wrapping their heads around that notion, I find, and for good reason. First, in US culture the word "sexuality" is most often defined one-dimensionally, as "those things having to do with sex." What's more, the media's ubiquitous obsession with physical sex creates and perpetuates the presumption that people are sexual only if and when they are *having sex*. So, how could people be sexual just by "being"? And—huh?—how could a newborn possibly be sexual?

Except for sexuality, we take for granted that human beings are not simply the sum of their physical parts and that our bodies and behavior don't exist in isolation from the rest of us. To be alive is to be in a dynamic and interactive state: we perpetually think, feel, learn, sense, experience, relate, communicate, evaluate, decide, problem solve, and interact with other living beings and our environment—all at once. And we also inhabit a body and engage in a variety of behaviors that are shaped by these very thoughts, feelings, values, experiences, and interactions. To define ourselves simply in terms of the physical is to ignore the rest of our humanity and our "being."

Sexuality—a part of us that's literally built in at birth—is every bit as complicated and dynamic.[1] Let's do take it apart from a purely physical standpoint first. Even as adults, the majority of Americans probably don't fully appreciate that all people have both a sexual system *and* a reproductive system. Even though they overlap in significant ways, the two systems in fact function independently. Though babies won't be able to make babies for years, their sexual system—part of the sensory portion of the central nervous system—is already up and running at birth. Indeed, probably the first thing most baby boys do right after they're born is have an erection; that's the sexual system waking up to a totally different environment—bright/cool/dry/ open versus dark/warm/moist/cozy—along with the rest of the body. (One of my students insists that no, it's just the penis making sure it works.) Dr. William Masters, an ob-gyn and pioneering sexual researcher and therapist, used to have a running bet with his anesthesiologist that he could cut a baby boy's umbilical cord before it happened. He must have been mighty quick.

People often are shocked to learn something else about themselves—and their babies—as sexual people. Each day or night, at ninety-minute intervals during the brain's natural sleep cycle, starting *before birth*, penises become erect (my student insists that's to make sure they're still working), and in females, the vaginal walls release sexual lubricating fluid. Like all other cycles in our bodies—breathing, digestive, cardiac, menstrual, etc.—our sleep/sexual cycle is inherently a part of us. A baby boy or girl is in no way sexual in the same ways as adults, but he or she, by physical nature, is a sexual being nonetheless.

Beyond the physical, all children begin to learn about their sexuality in a social and psychological sense the very moment they are born. Stop and think for a minute about the first thing anyone ever said about you—It's a boy! It's a girl!—and when and how they said it. Imagine, all eyes in the delivery room *right there* the very second those genitals are out. Clearly that part of us is ultra-important to the people who welcome us into the world; let's not think for a moment that babies don't eventually read that message and start paying extra attention *right there* to discover what all the fuss is about.

As I write, our daughter-in-love (I so prefer that to "daughter-in-law") is pregnant with our first grandchild. It's so exciting. Everyone of course asks right away, "Do you know what they're having?" "Yes," I sometimes answer. "I'm really happy to say it's a human! There was some concern at first it might be a platypus, but no, it's definitely a human." People always laugh, but there's a serious side to my quip as well. We're so quick in American culture to relegate children to one side or the other of the gender divide—did you know even bingo sets for children now come in "princess" and "frog prince" versions? (Growing up, my friends and I hadn't a clue there was a *boy way* to play bingo and a *girl way* to play bingo; we just loved yelling "bingo," you know, in a gender-neutral sort of way.) I wish we could get to know children—and grow children—more fully and purely as brand-new humans, with the emphasis right off the bat on how boys and girls are the same, not how they're different.

So here's my first point about affirmation and sexuality: your children have been going to "sex and gender school" since the very second they were born, and no matter their age, they still are. (And here in the United States we think that "sex-ed" starts with a film in the fifth grade about periods or wet dreams!) Sexuality is as much a part of their ongoing development as the acquisition of language, motor skills, communication, and self-esteem. And think about how much deliberate and considered attention we pay to those things. Our children's sexuality is no different: once we fully acknowledge it, we can fully nurture it. This chapter will help you watch it evolve seamlessly in front of your eyes and help you anticipate what will likely come along next that will need your attention.

For example, here's a quick way to literally "see" your children's emerging sexuality. One day soon, go and take a fresh look around your children's rooms. Take it all in, including the furnishing and accessories, what's in the drawers and closets and on the walls and the floor, and even under the bed. Then mentally remove what you see—or *smell*, as some parents are quick to point out to me—that most definitely or very likely wouldn't be there if she or he were the other gender. (In many cases, it might be way easier to count the items that would be left.)

All the stuff you just removed is probably a pretty accurate reflection of what your kids have been absorbing in gender school since day one about what it means to be a girl or to be a boy. If you examine it as a social scientist might, what does each item say about who boys and girls are or are not supposed to be, what they like and don't, what's deemed appropriate for them, or not? What do they seem to cherish most—what values, traits, activities, assets, goals, heroes, role models, music, books, electronics, games, and clothing—and how have they come to treasure these things? What and who have been most influential? How much of what you see is innate, do you think, and how much is the product of environment and learning? What are your children gaining, and what might they be losing, because of the gender roles—which are really gender *rules*—that culture and circumstance impose?

And how do you feel about whatever you've discovered?

Developmental Highlights

I hope it's clearer how sexuality is a central and integrated component of the whole self—arguably the most central, since it's the very first part of us to be acknowledged by the world we came into; literally everything else in life comes *after* and is built on top of it. Described in the sections below is a sketch of what parents can expect as children's and adolescents' sexuality evolves in the context of their ongoing development. It's meant to provide a general developmental profile and to highlight key themes, important transition points, "red flags," and general tips. We'll circle back to more specific how-to skills in the chapters to follow.

A proviso: most readers of this book are not parents of infants, which is where this profile begins. It's useful reading for all parents, though, since it highlights how development unfolds in a continuous spiral, with one stage building on and revisiting the last. Also, as you read through, don't think for a second that somehow you blew it if you didn't do or say something at a particular age or stage: *It's never too early and never too late to support healthy sexual development*. Please remember my friend Frank from the previous chapter, who caught up to his daughter's development in a flash when she was fourteen years old.

And some reassurance: I included much of what you'll find below in *Sex and Sensibility*[2] more than ten years ago, when the "tween" marketing campaign was just gaining steam, and when, overall, the boundaries separating the child and adults were much less porous. It matters not, though: Development is development, and it proceeds today pretty predictably in the same ways as always. Who children and teens are at each stage—regardless of what they may be encouraged to do that's beyond their years—hasn't changed at all; when profound change happens around them, it changes their lives, but not their developmental capacities. It's good to keep that in mind in deciding what they are—and are not—ready for.

Birth to Age Two

Intimacy. During children's earliest years, whether parents are consciously aware or not, they provide the foundation for children's later sexual life. If you think about it, the pleasure and comfort infants come to associate with their parents' strong arms, loving voice and touch, and physical warmth and presence provide their very first and most important lessons about the joys of physical and emotional intimacy. One of the best ways I've found, in fact, to explain the connection between intimacy and sex is to ask my students— as young as eleven and as old as eighteen—to reminisce about the experience of cuddling with parents and grandparents. (I'm always so happy to discover that many still do cuddle, even the older ones, including boys.) I ask them to recall the amazing physical and emotional feelings that fill us up so quickly when we are that physically close to someone we love and cherish and who loves and cherishes us. The collective list they make is very long, and very wonderful. That's it right there, I tell them, the unbelievable and nearly instantaneous power of human physical contact.

Body. Adults also support and affirm children's healthy development by showing approval and acceptance toward their bodies (including the sexual parts and their nearby neighbors, the urinary and digestive openings) and their functions and products. Every time we give a bath or change a diaper we send potent messages about sexuality, both nonverbally—through our body tension, tone of voice, and facial expressions—and verbally, in the things we say and the words we choose. If we can sustain the same even, matter-of-fact tone and approach toward these parts and functions as we do all others, we help them accept the sexual parts of their bodies as fundamentally positive and part of an integrated whole.

On the other hand, when caretakers suddenly tense up whenever a baby or toddler happens to touch his or her genitals, or show extreme disgust or discomfort toward a messy bowel movement or a sudden erection, or use babyish or silly names for penises, vulvas, urine, or feces, rather than the proper words we use for other body parts or products, they communicate that these parts are somehow separate and apart, bad or inferior, or even fraught with danger. Anytime sexual parts are defined or treated as separate and "other," it leaves the impression that sexuality is different and disconnected from the rest of life. The most important and most powerful message of all is that our sexuality is the same.

Imagine the power of simple acknowledgment in saying, "I see you like to rub your vulva because it feels good."

For some parents I know just the idea of thinking that last sentence, let alone saying it, sends waves of panic down their spine. When I ask why, they usually express the worry that being "too" direct or positive with young children might create "too much" interest in "sex" at "too early" an age. To my well-trained ears, I tell them, that sounds an awful lot like Puritan speak (it's the word "too" that gives it away), reinforced by a dose of American-style confusion over the difference between encouraging healthy sexuality development and encouraging "sex."

Overlapping growth and development. Another way to more easily integrate sexuality into the concept of a child's overall development is to remember that children and adolescents, unlike adults, are in a rapid state of growth and change in four different ways all at once: intellectual, physical, social, and emotional. Since sexuality is a component of children's organic selves, "sexual development" and learning are also part intellectual, physical, social, and emotional.

For example, babies, as we know, love to touch and explore their bodies inside, outside, and all over. That's because the human body is their first classroom, their starting place for all *intellectual* learning and discovery, because it is literally so close at hand. At first they explore at random; wherever the fingers or hands land determines the lesson for the moment. Inevitably, of course, fingers will find their way to a sexual part, prompting brand-new— and rather startling—discoveries. *Note to self:* "Oh my! Touching that part feels *really* different from pulling on my earlobe or rubbing my nose! And not only that, it feels *really* good, too! It would be lovely to happen upon *that* fun and interesting part again." Luckily, advancing *physical* maturation will allow for greater muscle control and coordination, and exploration can become more self-directed and purposeful. Small wonder that for many babies these particular anatomical parts, whenever they happen to be accessible (one of the great perks of graduating from diapers to big-girl pants), will become destinations of choice again and again and again.

In the self-directed and purposeful department, I'm thinking about my little cousin. When she was three she always wanted to go in Grandpa's car, not Grandma's car, whenever she had a choice. It got to the point where Grandma started to feel a little hurt. Finally she asked her why, and Molly said, "'Cause, silly, the straps on the car seat in Grandpa's car always make my 'tickle place' feel really good." (When she was a little younger, she discovered her vagina while bathing and said, "Mommy, I found a pocket!")

As part of normal maturation, infants and toddlers gradually develop the ability to read social cues and interpret their meaning. The expressions on Mom's or Dad's face, for example, provide a new level of learning about themselves and their bodies: "Hmmm. People look at me differently when I pull on my penis than when I pull on my earlobe. Oh, I get it! Different parts of my body have different kinds of *social* meaning. How fascinating!" Over time, if the reactions they notice are consistently positive and accepting, they will likely come to associate their sexual parts and the pleasurable sensations they provide with *emotional* feelings, such as pride and happiness. On the other hand, if the attention feels consistently disapproving, they may feel confused (how could such good feelings be bad?) or even guilty or ashamed (maybe *I'm* bad, because I like doing something that Mom or Dad—or Grandma or Grandpa or my nanny—thinks is bad).

So there you have it: intellectual, physical, social, and emotional growth and change interacting to inform and shape the course of sexual development.

Ages Two to Five

Language. Repeat after me: penis, foreskin, scrotum, testicles, vulva, clitoris, labia, vaginal opening, urethra, urine, urinate, anus, bowel movement, buttocks. Not quite yet everyday words? Repeat after me: penis, foreskin, scrotum, testicles, vulva, clitoris, labia, vaginal opening, urethra, urine, urinate, anus, bowel movement, buttocks. Not yet? Repeat. Then repeat them again five times a day for the next five days (or make it ten times a day for ten days, depending) and I guarantee they'll become what they've always been: meaningless letters strung together to create words just like ear, eye, nose, breathe, smile, mouth, navel, foot, and walk. (Okay, okay. Those were a lot shorter and easier to say and spell, especially for a child, but don't even go there. Have you ever heard a three-year-old pronounce the word "laminate"? Or "esophagus"? Well, I have. "Urinate" is a piece of cake.)

But, you may say, what if my daughter were to repeat those words in front of my mother, or worse yet, at school? Time to ask, methinks, what's wrong with this picture, and whose needs are we here to meet anyway? Here's the truth, in the service of raising sexually intelligent children in the twenty-first century: grandparents and others will just have to get over it (or we'll just have to get over their disapproval). It can be done. I remember once when my mother and mother-in-law—born within days of each other in 1914—were over for dinner and one of my young sons took the occasion to announce, "I'm really proud I'm a boy!" "Why is that?" someone asked. "Because when a man and a woman have sexual intercourse, the sperm gets there first!" My mother, by this time well educated about developmentally appropriate needs and behavior, said simply, "Please pass the peas," to which my mother-in-law replied, "Buttered or plain?"

As for fears about the playground or lunch table—*Horrors! Kids who actually know something for a change spreading it around at school!*—understanding child development can help in the commonsense department. By the time children are old enough to form the thought, "Cool! I think I'll tell everyone at school," they're also mature enough to grasp the concept of privacy (e.g., they know to close the bathroom door, keep their clothes on in public, knock if a door is closed). A simple request, delivered in an even tone of voice— "Please keep this information private, since these are parts of us we keep private"—will likely do the trick.

Privacy versus secrecy. I know a fourth grader whose mom, determined that she know the facts, bought her a book when she was younger about "stuff," as the girl called it. But before settling in to read with her, the mom very deliberately got up to close and lock the door. It was such a dramatic aberration, the girl remembered that part of the story most clearly, and not much of anything about the book. Afterward, her mom told her firmly, "Don't tell this information to *anyone*."

Recognizing clearly—and teaching our kids—the difference between secrecy and privacy can help avoid the unnecessary confusion and negativity, and the slight case of fright, my young friend was left with. And you know, what's the big secret anyway? So what if your very young child points to each and every person in the very long "ten or fewer" line at the supermarket and announces, oh, say, fairly loudly, which one has a vulva and which one has a penis? Go ahead—name one adult in the entire store who didn't know that already. Well, actually, since many adult women don't know the difference between their vagina (on the inside) and their vulva (on the outside), I might have to amend that remark. But, hey, isn't it time they knew?

Curiosity. Speaking of body parts, young children are purposely hardwired to notice *difference,* because it prompts curiosity and, thereby, the acquisition of knowledge. Body-part differences between boys and girls and men and women are no exception, and often invite very intense interest. My favorite story along these lines is about a little girl who happens to notice a little boy urinating at the edge of some trees. "Wow!" she says to him. "Where did you get that? What a neat thing to bring along to a picnic!" (I wonder if that's what Freud meant by "penis envy.") Children's natural curiosity about body differences is definitely something to encourage; bathing young siblings together or showering with parents (who are comfortable) are great vehicles. For households composed of people of the same gender, making a point of diapering or bathing your next-door neighbor's baby with your young child's help, or reading one of the lovely children's picture books on this topic together is just as helpful. Besides, when young children begin to ask questions about their origins, it's oh-so-helpful—for them and for us—if they've got some basic ideas about everybody's basic parts. It's hard to learn about multiplication without a working knowledge of addition.

Setting limits. Part of nurturing is setting appropriate limits around children's sexual curiosity, interests, and behaviors. We don't want our children masturbating inappropriately in public places (masturbation, in the original Greek, by the way, means "to defile oneself"; okay if we call it "self-pleasuring" instead?) or pointing out who has penises and who has vulvas at will, or inviting the whole neighborhood over to play doctor. All of these situations are best handled by recognizing that two separate needs are at stake in these kinds of situations (affirmation and setting limits), and that each requires a two-part response.

Saying something like the following will do the job: "You really enjoy touching your genitals. I'm sure that feels good. *And* [not "but"] you're a big girl now, so let's talk about some places where you can enjoy doing that in private." "You've learned a lot about people's genital parts. *And* people consider those parts private, so let's talk about this at home when we're alone." "You kids look like you're really curious about what boys' and girls' bodies look like. *And* when we have company in our house we keep our clothes on. So let's put them back and do something fun downstairs." (Or in this last example, you could just turn around and leave. Once their curiosity is satisfied, they'll get bored and come downstairs on their own.)

Ages Six to Nine

Six- to nine-year-olds are increasingly out and about beyond home, family, and school. Though very much still children, they have become much more rational beings. Within the confines of certain well-defined limits, they are capable of logical ideas, independent thinking, and responsible action. Life is no longer mostly play and focused moment to moment on their immediate needs, and they are put to the task of increasingly serious and structured learning in more formal school environments.

Curiosity. Children in early elementary school continue to ask questions about similar topics as before, but in more sophisticated ways. They often circle back to questions about reproduction—how babies are made, how they develop, and how they are born—and they may need to hear it all again and again before they get it all straight in their minds. They may also want more pointed information about sexual intercourse and how it happens, and might even ask if they can watch. That's a request, never fear, that has everything to do with their still very concrete approach to learning, and nothing to do with budding voyeurism.

By the end of first grade (I used to say second) most children will have heard sexual terms or references on the playground, around the neighborhood, from older siblings and cousins, on the Internet, over the radio, in movies, or on TV. (Recently I asked a group of fourth graders where they learned what they know about sex. Three of them said at the same time, "The dentist's." The dentist's? "Yes," they explained. "It's all over the magazine covers in the waiting room!") Some of these examples weren't even on the list five to ten years ago; even on network TV now, where shows with more "adult" content are still confined to later hours in the evening, their "sexy" promos aren't. Though many of these media references whiz right by younger kids, just the exposure itself connects them directly and artificially to an adult level of sexuality, and a grossly distorted one at that, they can't begin to understand and shouldn't have to. It's a time for strict and very deliberate supervision of their access to media in all forms, most especially the Internet and any and all electronic devices that can access it. *Whatever we can control, we should control.*

Six to nine is a stage when we want to work especially hard at *getting there first*, because it's the time when children first begin to construct an understanding of sexuality beyond the mechanics of reproduction. Their peers play a huge role in this—especially in American culture—because many adults send signals that they're not available yet to be a resource. Kids always know something's up if adults aren't talking, which only heightens their sense of curiosity, but also causes them to take it elsewhere. So, it's not at all unusual for sex or sexiness to pop up in conversation among early elementary–age kids, particularly at school and out of the earshot of adults.

Inviting conversation with your kids around playground chatter is a great place to start if you're ready to take this bull by the horns. No matter what other kids at school are talking about, encourage your children to bring it all home, so you can add your adult voice and perspective to the mix. You may need to get yourself shock proofed first: accessibility to sexual language and other content is so easy and widespread today that if your seven- or eight-year-old child came home today and asked, "Daddy, what's 'S and M'?" it wouldn't surprise me. (Was that a shock wave that just went through you? Look for pointers in the next chapter on how you might answer questions that seem wildly out of range.) Remind yourself that it's *just talk*; in itself it's not harmful, especially if you and your kids get in the habit of keeping open communication. And please remember that sex has been a hot topic of conversation on the playground since at least the 1950s, when I was in grade school. The specifics of what kids talk about today may be very different, but not *that* they talk.

This part is especially important: some of the most vital conversations with six- to nine-year-old children are less about *what* other kids are talking about than *how* they're talking about it. Be sure to ask your children about the "how" and "why" of playground banter, not simply the content, and give your best guidance about that, too. Here are some questions you might try out: When this subject comes up, are other kids giggly? Serious? Joking around? Acting secretive or even "naughty"? What kind of words do they use? Do kids who know more seem to get a lot of attention? Does anyone ever tease other people about what they don't know, or brag about what they do know? Do boys and girls talk equally as much, and in the same or different ways? Do people look comfortable? Uncomfortable? Does anyone ever try to use this topic to make another child feel bad? Are any "truth or dares" involved? How do boys and girls talk about or treat each other during these conversations? Are there adults around? Do they notice? Get involved? Do kids ever wait until adults are out of range to talk about sexuality? Why is that, do you think?

These kinds of questions tap into the really powerful but unspoken lessons six- to nine-year-old (and older) schoolkids teach each other every day about sex and gender. When parents invite children to bring home these experiences and observations, they create rich opportunities for reinforcing the ideas, attitudes, and values *they* want their kids to connect to sexuality. They give us the chance to say things like, "You know, sex is a serious subject, and it's important to look and sound serious when we speak about it," or "Some kids like to use sexual words to make other kids feel uncomfortable. What you overheard today is a really good example. Let's think about what you could say or do if someone said that to you."

Conversations like these also make crystal clear the difference between "telling kids about sex" and "talking with kids about sexuality." One approach provides information, while the other provides nurturing. As I wrote back in Chapter 1, nurturing around sexuality merely teaches the same kind of "life lessons" parents attempt to teach children every day around everything else. The two examples in the last paragraph aren't about "sex," but about helping kids learn *good ways to think and communicate* about sex.

When "life lessons about sexuality" come from other children rather than adults, they become the only strategies and approaches children know. Many, as a result, will come to associate sexuality—fundamentally—with joke-making, embarrassment, disrespect, discomfort, social power, name-calling, intimidation, and/or sexism, and those impressions may shape their behavior and their relationships *for years to come.* (I kid you not—not a minute after I added those italics, the phone rang and I got pranked by a girl who sounded thirteen-ish. "Hello," she said, while her friends laughed hysterically in the background. "I like boobies. Do you like boobies?" I rest my case.) As almost any high school teacher can tell you, many adolescents bring these very same ways of thinking and communicating right along with them into the high school scene and beyond.

One final point: I've become aware in the past few years that, more and more, older siblings (and cousins) seem to be taking it upon themselves to "teach the little kids" about things sexual. Whether they're showing off, goofing around, using younger children to score social points with their friends, or actually trying to help them get a leg up on sexual knowledge, it's almost never a good idea. As we've said, framing sexual information for younger children in a carefully constructed way is usually way more important than any facts given, assuming that the information is even accurate. This is another good thing to get ahead of. I would advise telling older siblings, etc., up front, "Thanks, but no thanks. The adults in the family need to handle this one."

Gender. As teachers and parents have long observed, six- to nine-year-olds tend to gravitate increasingly toward same-gender activities and relationships. Though many people view this dramatic shift as normal and "natural" at this age, I'm not convinced it's quite that simple or organic. I think there are some pretty powerful cultural influences at work.

By the early elementary school years, children have already absorbed some very particular "rules" about gender from American culture. They know, for example, that males and females are supposed to be "opposites," because that's how we in American society constantly refer to one another. Marketers, intent on creating male and female versions of practically everything, as if we have practically nothing in common, have been conditioning them for years to believe that there's a boy way to do things and a girl way to do them, too. They've also "caught" the idea from peers, advertisers, and media images—and sometimes parents and other adults—that there is a *right way* and a *wrong way* to "do" gender and, most important, that being the *right kind* of boy or girl is ultra-important. That's an awful lot of pressure. It makes perfect sense they would want to circle the wagons with same-gender peers, to learn best from one another how to become the very "best" boys and the very "best" girls they can possibly be.

Parents and teachers can do their very best to actively encourage girls and boys to sustain good friendships and positive, relaxed interactions with one another throughout the elementary school years. (I would say some of the happiest and healthiest kids I know in high school are those who have really good, long-standing friends of both genders.) That's probably the most effective way to diffuse the gender "rules" that fuel the tendency toward strict, self-imposed gender segregation. After all, children ultimately live out their lives in a coed world, and for most of them, the intimate relationships they form with the other gender will be central to a healthy and satisfying life. It truly does not serve them to think of each other as "opposites," or an entirely different species ("Ooooh, cooties!"). Parents and teachers can also take a more direct approach, by actively challenging the gender rules in American society that promote the idea that how we enact our gender—and the degree to which we approximate someone else's idea of the "right kind" of boy or girl—somehow determines our worth as human beings.

I think a lot about what the world today might look like if our society, and others, cherished the idea of nurturing the "right kind" of human beings instead.

"Gay." It's often during kindergarten or first grade (I used to say second) that the word "gay" begins to surface in children's conversations, usually when adults are somewhat at a distance, such as on the playground or the school bus, during recess, or at the lunch table. Though the concept is becoming more familiar to them, young children's life experiences around the word "gay," and with the idea that some people *are* gay, vary enormously.

Some children, of course, are raised by gay parents, or know that other people in their immediate family—or in their family's larger circle of relatives, friends, or acquaintances—are gay. To them, "gay" just *is*; it's a natural part of their social landscape. For other young children "gay" is a word they're simply curious about because they've heard other people use it and they enjoy learning the meaning of new words. Another child may have attended a gay-rights rally or heard a clergyperson say that being gay is wrong. Some have heard classmates arguing at the lunch table about whether gay people can get married, or trying to figure out if kids really can have two mommies or two daddies. Still others are confused about "gay" because they hear some children use the word as a verbal weapon or a "playful" insult and they have no idea why, or because "fag" and "gay" seem to mean the same thing, but "fag" is a bad word and "gay" is an okay word. They also know that boys might be called gay or fag when they're "acting like girls," but not girls when they're "acting like boys." And some kids aren't paying attention to any of it. Now, picture all these kids playing and jabbering at one another on the same playground on the same afternoon.

An ever-increasing number of lesbian, gay, bisexual, and transgender people are visible in American life, and their reality and their stories are gradually becoming, in ways big and small, part of *everyone's* social and cultural landscape. Truthfully, in many families and schools, the kids are way ahead of the adults in grappling with these changes, because they have to; they walk around on this new and potentially confusing landscape every day. Why, I think we should ask, are so many adults still standing out on the perimeter of these discussions instead of leading them?

I think the reason has everything to do with the basic theme of this chapter: that "gay" has something to do with sex. The narrow way we define sexuality in American culture—as those things having to do, literally, with sex—leads parents and schools to conclude that talking to kids about "gay" means talking to kids, literally, about gay sex. Again, we miss the forest for the tree. How to frame this topic (and others adults shy away from for similar reasons) in human terms, and not purely physical or sexual terms, is the theme of the next chapter.

All of this discussion is way too academic for the young people in our lives who are *right now* in the process of discovering they themselves are lesbian, gay, bisexual, or transgender. Their basic needs—for affirmation, information, clear values and limits, and anticipatory guidance—are no different from any other child or adolescent. But as a culture, we often create enormous obstacles and great psychic pain for these particular youngsters, especially when we think, act, and talk as if they aren't part of the social and cultural landscape at all. And that's the most damaging form of *disaffirmation* I can think of. So, let's all of us figure out a way to bring "gay" in from the playground, and adults in from the perimeter. More about how to do that in Chapter 8.

Grade by Grade by Grade

Most children age four to seven—unless they're exposed to adult-oriented media or spend a lot of time with other kids who've had lots of exposure— have an intermittent, curiosity-driven interest in sexuality and reproduction. They're also not much inclined to care about what their peers or media have to say about the subject. Around the age of eight, though, many children's interests can start to broaden fairly rapidly, as their social and intellectual development shifts into higher gear, and as peer and media influence begin to factor in to a much larger extent. Teachers and parents will likely see many changing dynamics as kids move forward from grade to grade in school. Here are some "nutshell" observations.

Third Grade

As I like to say, second grade is an important year for sexual development, mostly because it's the year before third grade. Parents of children under eight are wise to know that an important shift is coming, since interest in sexuality often heightens significantly in later elementary school—if not for their own daughter or son, then certainly for many children he or she interacts with. Forewarned is forearmed: what a good reason to open up the subject of sexuality in some way with your child by the end of the second-grade year, if you haven't already. (It's kind of like my advice to late fifth graders that *everyone* should come back to school next year wearing deodorant from day one; why be sorry?) This way, you'll have identified yourself as "askable" and approachable when the topic kicks into higher gear.

Playground banter about sexual language seems to increase exponentially among some eight-year-olds, but almost everyone is part of the experience. Though it's certainly tempting to blame the media for this turn of events, interest in things sexual at this age is logical and really quite predictable. My older son was eight in the early 1980s, long before the hypersexualization of American popular culture. He came home that year from school with some real doozies, including terms such as "pemp" (meaning "pimp"), "prostitute," "azho" (meaning "asshole"), "bases," and "blow up." This last one gave me real pause, I admit, and I finally decided that until he got it right, I wasn't obligated to explain it. (By the time he did, though, I had gotten myself ready.)

Children's behavior is always best understood in the context of overall development. The minds of middle to late elementary school children are newly able to grasp the concept of "society," beyond the confines of their own immediate social world. For the first time, they get a sense of the invisible thread or glue that binds together people, values, and institutions, not unlike what binds their family, school, or community, but bigger, more complex, and much less concrete. They also can conceptualize "future" much farther out in front of them than previously, and can visualize acting in it more realistically as more grown-up children, adolescents, and even to a degree, as adults. (Please note, these are the exact developmental attributes that led marketers to select age eight as the bottom end of the "tween" marketing niche.) Figuring out how this larger social, economic, cultural, and political universe works, and how they will eventually fit themselves into it, becomes one of the grown-up challenges middle to late elementary school children begin to shoulder and carry with them into adolescence.

As many a savvy fourth, fifth, and even third grader already understands, sex is one of the things that makes American society tick. After all, if you were a Martian who had just landed in American popular culture, wouldn't you categorically conclude that, too? At some point for young children, random but constant exposure to sexual content and innuendo abruptly coalesce into a new level of interest, and given the developmental imperative of the age, figuring out how society works *sexually* as well becomes a sudden and pressing priority.

Keep in mind, too, that this new level of interest is far removed from the mechanistically oriented concerns about origins and reproduction that engage younger children. The focus here is more on sex per se, that is, on sexual behavior and those things connected to it. Children this age are becoming aware that people "do it," and it's the "doing" part itself that has them fascinated and often disgusted, all at the same time—which for most children, of course, only heightens the interest.

In most schools, especially elementary schools, children know that "sex talk" is taboo, so they most often confine it to when and where they think they won't be overheard. Sometimes I have to reassure my students repeatedly that they won't get into trouble if they ask a certain question or say a certain word—even in sexuality class. What an awful message! Parents do well by their children when they become advocates for responsive and truly age-appropriate sexuality education (not the same thing at all as *puberty* education) beginning at least in third grade, so that teachers are more likely to receive encouragement and training to become allies in getting children off to a healthier start.

Fourth Grade

I've noticed for years that nine-year-olds are especially interested in learning about fetal development. Since children's interests in sexual topics mirror the larger developmental issues in their lives, fourth-grade fascination with growth and development in utero reflects the anticipation of their own coming "gestational period." They're also suddenly curious about bodies in a more personal kind of way, especially how people's bodies look when their clothes are off. They practically jump into my lap when I get to the page in my favorite book for upper elementary kids—Robie Harris's *It's Perfectly Normal*—which shows a range of bodies and how they're shaped. Children are palpably excited and relieved to see how easily their own body types fit in. What an important opportunity that is for kids on the brink of sexual development in a culture where marketers will constantly tell them that their bodies are *not okay*. Even sexual parts are now a target: the number of women, and men, who undergo genital surgery is rapidly on the increase (though the numbers are still relatively small), as more people—probably due to exposure to pornography—accept the notion that sexual parts, too, must meet certain standards of perfection if one is to be an acceptable partner. On top of all the extra sexual pressures on teens and young adults today, some are already adding "genital self-image" to the list. This will be an important issue for us to get ahead of.

It's clear that many fourth graders are the product of years of missed opportunities for age-appropriate sex and reproduction education. Consider the following anonymous questions, gathered from fourth-grade students: Why do men have penises and girls have vaginas? If you were born a boy, can you turn into a girl? Why do kids sometimes talk with kids about things they want to know, but never with a grown-up? Why does sex (I don't know what it is) cause children? What does "reproduction" mean? Where do babies come out of? Why do people's bodies change? What do babies' private parts look like?

Other questions make clear that fourth graders have been paying attention to sexual information and attitudes for years: Why is it assumed that "sex" is a bad word? Why are people scared to say "penis" and "vagina"? Why do kids sing and make up rhymes about private parts? Why do people make such a big deal about "doing it"? How come you never really are allowed to talk about it freely? Why does it get so important when you become a teenager? What does it mean to "blow someone"? Why do men find rape and harassment "nice"? Why do kids and adults make fun of gay people and lesbians? Who invented "fuck," "shit," "damn," "hell," and "bullshit"? How come people like seeing and making "sexy" movies? Why do they talk about their private life?

Fourth graders are also clearheaded and fair-minded on issues about which older students sometimes have blind spots. They have a keen sense of fairness about demeaning and disrespectful behavior and are uncommonly receptive to conversations about sexual labeling and bullying. Some are just beginning to test the power of sexist language with one another—"bitch," "'ho," "slut," "wimp"—and they have the brainpower to really understand an adult's explanation of why and how that language is unfair and hurtful. With continual reinforcement at home and at school, I'm convinced they would be less prone to carry this language—and the attitudes it conveys—into middle school social life.

Many at this stage are also beginning to emulate adolescent culture in their dress, hairstyles, makeup, accessories, language, and music. As we've said, just as teenagers have been recast in the image of young adults, and preteens as little teenagers, late elementary–age children are being encouraged to look and act like little grown-ups and to want the things that grown-ups (supposedly) want. The pressures on children and their parents can be enormous.

Late elementary school is the time for parents to take this not-yet-raging bull by the horns. Children not yet in the throes of adolescence still accept and expect that their parents will set limits around their behavior. Even if they don't especially like it, they know they are obliged to defer to adult authority. And the truth is, limits make them feel safe and cared for, despite the temper tantrums they may throw. *Now is a great time to set the stage for the adolescent years,* not by laying down the law or establishing who's boss, but by making it clear that parents have certain responsibilities you take and will always take very seriously. Here's the underlying message they need: "As the adult in our relationship, I will make certain decisions when it comes to your physical, social, and emotional well-being. You may not always like them, and in fact sometimes I'll make mistakes and underestimate or overestimate your ability to safely make your own decisions. But I will always try to be fair and realistic, I will always give you my reasons, and I will always ask for your input."

Parents would be very wise, too, to set up a supportive network with other parents, whether through grade-level meetings at their children's school or, more informally, by actively getting to know the parents of their children's friends. This is absolutely the best strategy I know to keep marketers from turning children into "tweens." Parents can decide together on guidelines for setting appropriate limits around socializing and other activities, remembering that uniform agreement isn't at all necessary: the exact limits each family sets are not as important as the strong, unambiguous message from all parents that it's appropriate and necessary to set them.

Routine communication among parents can also reduce children's ability to pit them against one another (one of their strongest suits): "But Sally's mom lets *her* do that!" Movies, music, TV, screen time, e-mail, texting, social networking, Internet use, sleepovers, bedtime, purchases, allowances, supervision, clothing, shoes, makeup, and so forth are all important and helpful topics for conversation. Other parents can also share strategies that work well. A woman in my recent class had a great one: "Here's what I tell my kids when they're badgering me to buy or allow them to do something: 'If you want an answer right now, it's a definite no. If you stop badgering me and give me a chance to think it over, the answer could be yes *or* no.' It works like a charm." Although parents cannot present a unified front on all issues (that would be impossible and far too heavy-handed), keeping in touch with one another helps clarify important developmental issues and highlights and reinforces everyone's affirmation and limit-setting roles.

Middle School

I am unabashedly in love with middle school kids. If you learn how to approach them just so, they are a joy (well, not *every* day) to teach. As a colleague describes them, children at this age are a cross between an automobile mechanic, a newspaper reporter, and a sponge: they want to know everything about everything, and they want to know it *now*. Obsessively fact- and detail-oriented, they insist on understanding how everything works, including their own bodies. Although they can be pretty embarrassed and giggly, their uncomfortable feelings are usually right on the surface, easy to identify, and not hard to diffuse. Also, since kids in this age group are gradually developing the brainpower required for thinking in abstract terms, they're eagerly drawn into—and terrifically excited by—discussions about complex ideas, controversies, and moral dilemmas. What wonderful opportunities for cultivating strong, clear values and critical thinking skills.

Also, from a cognitive, social, and psychological perspective, ten- to fourteen-year-olds are increasingly able to step outside themselves and think about their lives and their relationships with a much more grown-up point of view. They are ripe for looking at formal decision-making and problem-solving strategies. Moreover, even though sooner or later they will all be up to their knees in adolescent struggles over identity and separation issues, most are not yet even ankle deep; they are quite willing—even very publicly—to ask for adult input and guidance. The majority is also still clearheaded about risk-taking: they can tell you exactly what is good for you and bad, and through seventh grade at least, they're willing to make socially conservative statements about topics such as sex and drugs, even in front of their peers. In short, if you can get them to trust you and their classmates enough—and to sit still long enough—they're a sexuality educator's dream.

Double-digit status. I've included fifth graders among middle schoolers because in some schools that's the age when middle school begins. Although in most ways fifth graders are much more like children than early adolescents, their double-digit status can make them feel a cut above their younger schoolmates, as if they've crossed an important developmental threshold. Many of them have also begun to notice pubescent body changes in themselves or others, and they're consequently aware of boys and girls as different in new ways. A lot of girls, in particular, become almost painfully self-conscious at this age and are prone to over-personalize any mention of puberty or body changes. My goal in one recent class was to get two girls comfortable enough by the end of the period to come out from under the desk where they'd cloistered themselves! Boys generally are not seeing significant changes just yet and don't have any visible new attributes (e.g., developing breasts) to feel quite so self-conscious about.

The first time I held up a nondescript line drawing of a uterus and fallopian tubes in front of a group of fifth-grade girls, I was stunned to see at least five of them—mortified en masse—spontaneously cover their faces with their notebooks. To them, I finally realized, those were their own personal fallopian tubes I was showing the *entire* class! Parents, moms especially, are often just as dumbfounded by their fifth-grade (or slightly older) daughters' reticence, if not outright refusal, to talk about sexuality or even periods. If they've enjoyed a fun and pleasant history of easygoing and comfortable chats up to this point, they may feel mystified and even hurt or rejected by what is sometimes a very abrupt change. They might worry they've done something wrong or that there's something they're not doing right. Most likely, the sudden distance has nothing to do with them at all, and everything to do with normal, predictable physical and emotional changes.

The solution, as always, is for adults to recognize and put on the backburner their own reactions—real and understandable as they are—and have a look through the eyes of the child. In this case, a daughter's need for space and time enough to adjust and gain a renewed sense of developmental equilibrium is probably the issue. A parent can best help by affirming directly what the child is obviously feeling—"I can see that you're really not comfortable or interested in talking about this right now"—and letting her know that you'll be glad to talk again whenever she wants. She'll appreciate your attentiveness to *her* feelings and *her* needs, and she'll be way more likely to reconnect later on because she knows that her needs, not yours, come first. It's important to be aware of the difference, though, between *stepping back* for a period of time and *stepping out* of the picture altogether. We need to tell our kids directly that talking with them about sexuality is part of our job and that even without their prompting we'll be back.

Despite this sudden discomfort, it's not at all unusual for a few boys and girls at this age to start pairing up as couples, and the question of "Who likes who?" can become the hot topic for the entire grade. (Boys and girls in earlier grades sometimes pair up, too, but those kids are pretending they're growing up, whereas these kids know they really are.) Sometimes, especially with the lightning-fast communication that modern technology affords even younger kids today, things can get out of hand to the point of obsession. The rumor and gossip mill can take on near-epic proportions that can easily spill over into the school day, and teachers have to step in and call a halt to it.

If teachers—and parents—don't put brakes to this runaway train, it inevitably leads to hurt feelings and in group/out group power dynamics, as well as an artificial and restrictive definition of boy/girl relationships. Sadly, kids this age and older tell me they're afraid to be friendly toward certain boys or girls, because they're convinced other kids will spread the idea that they "like" each other. Imagine, as well, boys or girls in the midst of this scene, unable to relate or feel included at all, because they're beginning to question whether they might be gay. (The average age when people come out, first to themselves and then to others, has dropped significantly in recent years, so some will already know.) The unspoken heterosexism embedded in this "who likes who" frenzy—the assumption that everyone is and/or ought to be straight—can cause powerful feelings of isolation and invisibility, even at this tender age.

Fifth-grade "relationships" are very short-lived (except for two of my friends from grade school who've been together almost continuously ever since). They're simply a harmless kind of preparation and rehearsal for teenage life. Also, the experience of being called someone's boyfriend or girlfriend validates for yourself—and certifies publicly to your peers—that you're actually likeable in this new and important way. How exciting! Most commonly, the couple are content to confine their interaction to school time, the phone, and e-mail (if they're allowed access).

Parents may react with surprise or even alarm that sometimes a girl or boy at this age may want to ask someone out on a "date." (Slightly older kids sometimes will say they're "going out" with someone, which is ironic and funny since they most often don't actually go anywhere.) Making a big issue of the idea probably would be an overreaction, since children don't conceptualize dating in the same way as teenagers or adults. Instead, parents can use the situation to calmly initiate many opportunities (not all at once, of course) for affirmation, information giving, limit setting, and anticipatory guidance: What does it mean to you to go on a date? What kind of relationship should there be between people who date? What kind of dates—if any— are okay at your age? How about for older preteens? Older teens? How can you tell if someone is old enough or mature enough to go on a date? What is appropriate behavior on a date? Parents and kids can revisit these conversations time and again as "dating" takes on different meanings at different ages.

It's important for parents to think through their ideas and values in advance of these conversations, and to take care not to reinforce precocious behaviors by providing subtle encouragement ("Oh, isn't this cute!") or direct reinforcement ("Great! Let's go buy you something fantastic to wear!"). As marketers over the past decade have successfully attempted to redefine adolescence downward, I've become aware that an increasing number of parents today view formal "dating" among pre- and early adolescents as appropriate and even desirable, and a welcome sign of their children's social success. It's a reminder of just how vigilant adults today need to be about *who's educating us* about children and their needs.

Entering adolescence. A friend tells a very funny and revealing story about the day he discovered his eleven-year-old son had become an adolescent. The two of them were listening to the car radio, when a news story came on about the "morning-after pill." The father glanced over at his son a few times and noticed that each time the reporter said "morning-after pill" the boy seemed more and more confused. "But, Dad," he finally said, looking very earnest, "what do you use if you *do it* in the morning?"

The story didn't surprise me one bit. Sixth grade is a lot like third grade. It's one of those years when the antennae on top of a child's head abruptly shoot up two full notches instead of just one. Overheard words, phrases, facts, concepts, news items, and snippets of conversation that previously would have simply whizzed by suddenly begin to materialize on the child's radar screen. In fact, information is penetrating so rapidly at this age, I always joke that each sixth grader really needs his or her own personal sexuality tutor.

Twelve-year-olds I run into in the hallway often have a new question or two, and they nearly always begin with the words "Is it true that? . . ." Having overheard some brand-new nugget of information *this minute,* they just can't wait to check it out. To teach them, I seldom have to prepare so much as a tentative lesson plan: they'll eventually ask every question necessary for me to give them every piece of information I wanted to get across in the first place. And invariably, should we happen to leave something out, a student or two will catch me on the way out the door (or in the bathroom later in the day). Kids this age seem to instinctively know there's a great big puzzle of knowledge out there requiring assembly in their minds and that they need *all* the pieces to get it right. Again, this is how they think about *everything.* Why would sexuality be any different?

Their interests at this age extend way beyond reproductive facts and information about sexual behavior, since the issue of sexuality suddenly has become less academic and much more personal. Given the opportunity for freewheeling discussion, they will want to spend time talking about a large variety of topics. Changing bodies and the new feelings of privacy, modesty, and self-consciousness they provoke—especially for very early or very late developers—are hot topics. So are changing feelings and relationships with friends, family, and same- and other-gender peers.

As the school year proceeds, cliques, popularity, and the need to fit in begin increasingly to drive the social dynamic. Peer cruelty as a means of social control and dominance may rear its ugly head in powerful ways at this age—though parents and teachers report increasingly that these same dynamics now shape the lives of younger and younger elementary schoolkids as well. Add the unprecedented ease, reach, and lightning speed of communicating through e-mail, texting, and social networking (now available to an expanding number of middle school *and* lower school children) and these dynamics grow ever more worrisome and alarming. Much more on Internet use and abuse in Chapter 7.

Conversations around these issues are essential, especially for kids who don't easily fit the stereotypical mold of what's "in." As more boys and girls start to eye one another as potential romantic interests, and getting a boyfriend or girlfriend becomes a more widespread priority, navigating this new social terrain provides more grist for the rumor (and, hopefully, class discussion) mill. They'll also want to talk about the crude and sexist language that the genders use against one another and that the girls especially are bothered by. And of course, they're more than anxious to talk and ask questions about all the sexual content they've seen in movies and TV or on the Internet, and the chatter about sex they hear from one another.

Although later they will keep many of these same topics away from adult ears, at this stage, trusted parents and teachers are often welcomed happily as listeners, affirmers, and anticipatory guides. And in schools, where groups of kids can talk together, teachers can help them help one another, by normalizing common experiences ("Well, if others feel this way, maybe I *am* normal!") and boosting self-esteem. These are opportunities not to be missed.

One final observation: I often think of sixth and seventh grade as *the* pivotal years regarding kids' attitudes about sexuality, because they're exposed so quickly to so many new and different ways of thinking and talking about sex and gender. It can be a make-or-break time for many kids in developing healthy versus not-so-healthy attitudes and values they will carry with them into adolescence and even beyond. Adult input, I'm convinced, is the most decisive factor.

In the middle of the middle. Seventh grade is the perfect year for a formal, comprehensive, semester-long course in school on the broad topic of human sexuality. I've taught one for thirty-five years. A tad more comfortable and at home with their bodies (many have been experiencing changes for quite a while), seventh graders are still fairly close to and dependent on adults in their lives for guidance and support. Many are developing or refining fledgling abilities as abstract thinkers, and I'm hard-pressed to think of any sexual or gender-based topic they can't understand or critically analyze with help. It's simply a wonderful age for shaping healthy attitudes and building a broad base of knowledge as well as critical thinking, decision-making, and interpersonal skills. And the timing is perfect, since all of them are on the brink of fully entering adolescence.

As many of us still remember, seventh grade can be a very tough age socially and emotionally. Parents often describe these newly crowned teenagers as unbelievably self-centered. Many days they're so focused on their own needs, feelings, looks, insecurities, and perceived imperfections, they're almost impossible to please if not downright unfit to live with. They may bristle sharply at the way adults—especially their parents—speak to them or even look at them. They'll react with fury if they feel babied, snap shut like clams if adults pry, and may stop sharing things altogether if they're afraid we'll overreact or "catastrophize" their problems. It's also an age when peer approval and acceptance are probably never more important to achieve and never harder to come by. Just think, I tell parents, how hard it is for *you* to please them. Imagine what it must be like for them to come to school every day, desperately needing to please a room or grade full of kids who are all just as hard to please and live with as they are.

For young adolescents, this difficult stretch of time requires nerves of steel; for us, it requires patience and the knowledge and acceptance that this trial by fire is an unfortunate but necessary part of entering adolescence and beginning to take responsibility for themselves. As those of us who've watched our children live through this period remember well, there's very little parents can do to "fix" anything, but there's plenty to do in the way of listening, affirming, and helping their kids anticipate and know how to cope with the problems that will inevitably surface. Genuinely believing in them and their ability to conquer this stage may be the best support of all.

It helps, I think, to remember that we're probably *supposed* to feel relatively helpless and on the sidelines in these situations. From this point on, the views of their peers will carry infinitely more weight than ours about many things; they're now compelled to look to one another—not us—to affirm their basic acceptability and worth. No wonder the need for conformity, popularity, and loyalty to their peers peaks at this age; it speaks volumes about how desperate they are to find and create safe ground as they take their first precarious leaps away from us and our unyielding and unconditional love.

Young teens will have increasing opportunities to test their growing independence, as they begin to take all kinds of new risks, including sexual ones.

They may have their first serious crush and their first real sexual experiences. Holding hands, kissing, cuddling, and touching may become an occasional but important part of their social lives, and the experience of getting and giving sexual pleasure a new and powerful reality. From now on, their interest in sex will be prompted no longer by simple curiosity or external stimuli, but by internally based needs and desires. Self-pleasuring, now most often to the point of orgasm, increases and typically becomes the topic of playful banter (especially among the boys). In short, they become sexual beings in profound new ways.

Fifteen- to Eighteen-Year-Olds

Pulling in and away. By the end of the eighth-grade year, virtually everyone has entered full-fledged adolescence and is engaged in the hard psychological work of discovering his or her unique identity. I always say that you can just see it in their eyes one day. There's a sudden wariness or distance, or maybe just the slightest of veils, but it's unmistakable. They've pulled themselves inward and away from the surface. In part they're in hiding (they don't know yet who the "new real me" is, so it makes them feel too vulnerable to put themselves totally "out there") and in part they've simply got so much internal work to do that they have little extra energy to reach out and connect. Being "cool" sets in with a vengeance, and they wear it like armor: "If I'm cool, I'm invulnerable. If I act like nothing bothers me, then maybe nobody will bother me. If I seem to have everything together, maybe no one will guess I'm barely holding anything together." And it will be harder and harder for them to ask for help—even, and maybe especially, from trusted adults—since showing they need it would both blow their cover and defeat the purpose of proving they can do it on their own. Parents may find they are suddenly at arm's length.

As children become middle teens, they and their peers become the absolute creators of their social world, and increasingly their social world becomes their *real* world. It may look and feel as if we're being edged out of the picture, or even outright rejected ("You just don't understand *anything* about my life, so just leave me alone!"), but looks are deceiving. Our relationship with them has been downshifted, not downgraded, as pressing developmental imperatives increasingly make demands on their time, energy, and psyche. They know they can take our love for granted, and they only reject us precisely because they know they can. Don't think for a moment they've stopped caring, or needing and wanting both your acceptance and approval, or that they won't come back. Some of the most wrenching conversations I've had over the years have been with kids who are devastated because they disappointed their parents or violated their trust. They really do want to make us proud.

Adults can help most through these years by keeping a loving distance, being genuinely interested but not overly involved, and caring but not smothering, and by remembering that high school–age children need ever-increasing independence, but not total autonomy. There is still much for parents to do because there is much for adolescents to accomplish: completing their academics, cultivating unique talents, earning and learning to manage money, planning for their future, and fulfilling their personal, family, religious, and community obligations in increasingly adult ways.

As teens take on a greater number of adult responsibilities and characteristics, their needs for affirmation, information, clarity about values, limit setting, and anticipatory guidance take on multifaceted and complex new dimensions. If they (and we) adjust well to these new demands, by the latter high school years, when their adolescent angst may be in large measure resolved, they often reemerge as refreshingly real, approachable, and thoroughly appealing young adults. If we've done our jobs, in most cases just when we are enjoying them the most, we know we have to give them over to themselves.

Socially and sexually, during the high school years our roles as parents and teachers also remain crucial. It is self-serving and irresponsible just to say, "Oh well, I guess they know it all already." (Often we will have to convince them of the folly of that belief as well.) They will need a broad base of very practical sexual health information, and opportunities to work through embarrassment or discomfort and other barriers that may keep them from using it as needed. And they'll need help and support in understanding the relationship between sex and intimacy, or even that there is a relationship, since popular culture—and often peers—frame sex in purely physical terms.

As they become more sophisticated thinkers, older teens will rethink their sexual values and want to hear their peers think out loud about theirs—one of the best reasons of all for a high school human sexuality education program. Their social life outside of home and family will become increasingly active, but they'll continue to need the watchful eyes and skillful limit setting of adults, especially as alcohol (and other drugs) and driving become an escalating part of the picture. They will date (although the exact form will vary greatly from teenager to teenager, community to community, and school to school) and many will develop intense romantic relationships. Most will experience the awful and awesome pain of rejection and unrequited feelings; they'll need us to listen to, or at least respect, their anguish. Many will struggle mightily to differentiate infatuation from love, closeness from ownership, good sex from good relationships, intimacy from lust, conflict from battle.

Through it all, we can also help by clarifying "adulthood" in realistic and honest terms. Too often, in the eyes of teenagers and in society's depiction, an adult is someone who does "adult" things—driving, drinking, spending money, having sexual experiences. We can help them see that being an adult involves *how* we do things, not *what* we do. They will inevitably make some very good decisions and some very bad ones, and we may never know about many of them either way. But if we keep encouraging them to stay connected to us as anticipatory guides, we'll maximize the chances—and research confirms this—that they'll put off making major decisions, the ones that can most affect their health and their future, until they're secure and mature enough to make the right ones. The next few chapters will provide many practical suggestions for holding on and letting go in healthy balance.

5

Information:
Folding in the Facts

A comment on a high school girl's course evaluation a couple of years ago made my semester: "Thanks for folding in the facts instead of making them the point. Facts are only good if you know how to think about and use them." What a perfect stage-setter for Chapter 5.

American children and teens are literally bombarded with all kinds of information about sex. It's referenced almost everywhere in their lives, all the time. The poor quality of much of this information aside, the sheer quantity unnerves me more than anything, because it often leads them to conclude that they are sufficiently, if not extremely, well informed. What's more, older kids, seasoned teachers tell me, don't ask them nearly as many questions as they used to. It's just easier to "look it up on the Net."

The problem, of course, is that being *well informed*—that is, having lots of factoids, even if they're true—is not at all the same thing as being *well educated*. Tidbits picked up from here and there, no matter how numerous, do not an educated person make; information absorbed haphazardly—like a sponge soaks up water—fills crevices in the mind but can't provide a platform for making good decisions.

Being well educated about sex and sexual health is the opposite of haphazard. It's like an uncluttered desktop on your computer, where everything you need is stowed away in tidy and easily retrievable files. (My children, having seen the constant chaos on my desktop—I currently have seventy-four windows open in Firefox—will laugh out loud when they read that sentence.) Each file is filled with complete information—you may know nine really important things about HIV, but it's the tenth piece you don't know that could hurt you—and there's an automatic filter that screens for factual errors. Off in the corner is a file for "nice to know" facts; the "need to know" stuff is right in the center. And there's a built-in fail-safe search engine that takes you only to reliable sites.

There is also a folder, labeled "Academics," with thirteen ordered files of increasingly sophisticated knowledge, one for each year of school from kindergarten through twelfth grade, because that's how schools teach everything else, right? Setting in motion a spiral of learning—that builds in the basics early on and then gradually integrates more and more complex information going forward—is, of course, how young people would learn best about sexuality, too.[1]

As you've no doubt noticed, this is not the way things are done here in the United States. We hold on to the idea that there's a fixed quantity of sexual information adults need to keep close to the chest until we think the kids are ready, and then we can safely turn it over—whole! In short, we act more like guards and gatekeepers than educators. The equivalent of teaching math that way would be to keep arithmetic and multiplication a secret, and then start right out in fourth grade with fractions, or in eighth grade with algebra, or twelfth grade with calculus. We would know right away how nutty that would be.

Of course, hard as many adults may try to keep sex a secret, children, remember, have been going to sex and gender school since day one; it's not as if they grow up in a sexual vacuum. Every year from the ten- and eleven-year-olds I teach I hear vivid proof of just how much incidental information they're absorbing. Come with me to their first formal sexuality class, when

I ask them as a group to define the word "sex," and this typically is what you'll hear:

Sex is reproduction.
Sex is when the sperm meets the egg.
Sex is when the dick goes in the doughnut.
Sex is making a baby.
Sex is when a man sticks his thing in a girl's hole.
Sex is about love.
Sex is intercourse.
People do it for money.
Sometimes it's rape.

At first glance the students' answers may seem plausible and predictable—some even "cute." A deeper look, though, reveals equivalencies in the children's minds between things that are really quite different, for example, sex and reproduction; sex and vaginal intercourse; sex and heterosexuality; and sex and love (although, in truth, they can't for the life of them explain what a penis and vagina touching actually has to do with love). They're also aware that some people "do it" for money and that others are forced—concepts, understandably, they struggle with a lot.

To them sex is about particular body parts rubbing, eggs and sperm joining, and things men or boys do to women or girls. (Often they're not entirely happy with the verb "sticks" when they say it but can't think of how else to express it.)

The question makes many of them very uncomfortable—some can't even bring themselves to use words and resort to hand gestures instead—and there's a good bit of laughing, silliness, and joke-making. When asked why that's so, some will say, "Because sex is funny!"

Where to begin? What these students reveal is what they've learned and concluded about sexuality already, long before they enter a classroom. They teach us that unless we actively engage children in sexuality education well before fourth grade, from that point on much of it going forward is going to have to be *fundamentally remedial*.

Subsequently, teachers can help them unlearn and relearn—and re-sort, recategorize, and recontextualize—but very likely what they've learned first will stubbornly endure with far-reaching effects, since new information acquired going forward will be filtered, and understood, through this earlier lens. If you learn from a trusted friend when you're five, for example, that $2 + 2 = 6$, and nobody corrects you on that until you're nine or ten, you'll still think $6 + 6 = 14$, and $10 + 10 = 22$.

Imagine how differently a fourth- or fifth-grade class might proceed if all students came in already firmly understanding the following facts and concepts:

- ✓ Sexual behavior, or sex, is a special way that people bring their bodies close together. It gives people's bodies very warm and amazingly pleasurable feelings and under the best circumstances causes them to feel very close to each other.
- ✓ Sexual intercourse is a kind of sexual behavior, or a kind of sex, but not the only kind. It is a very powerful kind of sex because it can lead to making a baby. Sexual intercourse is something that two people choose to do together, not something one person does to another.
- ✓ Sexual intercourse and making a baby are not the same things. Sexual intercourse can lead to making a baby, but not always. Most of the time people choose to have sexual intercourse because they enjoy the feelings of pleasure and closeness they experience, not because they want to have a baby.
- ✓ People can have sexual experiences with people of their same gender or the other gender.
- ✓ Sometimes you may see people laugh or make jokes about sex or about their own or other people's sexual parts. That's because they feel embarrassed, not because sex is funny. Sex can be fun, but it can also be very powerful, so in this family, or this classroom, we try hard to look and sound respectful when we talk about this subject. People can talk about sex without feeling embarrassed, and even if they are embarrassed, they can control how they express those feelings.

✓ Sexual behavior can be misused. For example, sometimes people try to force other people to have sex. That is always wrong. Sometimes people let other people use their bodies for sex as a way to make money, but sex is supposed to be about caring for and about the other person, and enjoying being with each other in this special way.

So, How Could You Set That Kind of Learning in Motion?

I learned a very long time ago that if you want to know how to talk to kids about sex, the trick is to "listen first, and lesson-plan later." It's really that simple, especially if you're the parent of young children: just give out the message that you really want to hear and answer their questions—all of them—and they'll usually tell you *exactly* what they need and want to know. And you probably won't even have to tell them you're open to the dialogue; most of the time they just know. (Conversely, they usually can sense our reluctance, too.) You don't have to be perfectly comfortable or confident either, just willing to plunge in no matter what.

For thirty years, I've been asking parents the following: In your experience, at what age do children begin to ask questions about their origins, and what are the questions they typically ask? The consistency of parents' responses over time absolutely convinces me that there is a near universal and predictable sequence of questions young children are prone to ask—and answers they're specifically looking for—roughly between the ages of four and six, and that the sequence of these questions is directly related to the child's normal pace and progression of his or her cognitive development. No great surprise there, and yet another way of understanding that sexual development is not "different" but the same.

Age Four: Where Did I Come From?
Teachers of four-year-olds will tell you that for the very first time children begin to understand that they are physically separate from everything else in the world. Three-year-olds, for example, really do believe that everything and everybody around them disappears whenever they close their eyes. But fours

know better. "Separate" to a four-year-old means that he—and every other physical object in the universe—has distinct boundaries, as in, a clear beginning and a clear ending. That's the first developmental clue as to why many at this age so predictably ask, "Where did I come from?" Since everything and everyone has a clear beginning and a clear end, they reason, so must I! It's all about bookends: if you've had a four-year-old in your life, you know this is the age when they typically ask their first questions about death, too.

The timing of this question also has to do with time, literally. Time means very little to a three-year-old—it's way too abstract a concept. Show a photo of you and an older sibling to your three-old-daughter and she'll say something like, "Why aren't I in that picture, too?" The logical response, "It was before you were born," will make perfect sense to you, but I guarantee what she'll be thinking is, "Huh?" That's because there are two words in the sentence a three-year-old can't begin to comprehend: "born" and "before."

To a four-year-old, however, "before" is a piece of cake, because by then time is a working intellectual concept. So if we put it all together, what prompts the "Where did I come from?" question is something like this: "Oh, I get what you were saying, Dad, about that picture in the living room. After I was born I was *here*, but *before* I was born, I wasn't. So I must have been someplace else! Please tell me, Dad, where was I *before* I was *here*?"

Now, many parents will interpret the question, "Where did I come from?" (or its more generic version, "Where do babies come from?"), through their adult lens on the world, often projecting their worst fears: "Oh my God! I have to tell her about (adult) sex!"

I promise you this: your child is not asking about adult sex, isn't interested in adult sex, doesn't want to know about adult sex, in fact cares about it not one whit. What your child does care about in this case is simple *geography*: the question is literally about *where*. The answer, "Before you were born you were in a special place inside Mom's body called her uterus," will hit the mark perfectly. No sweaty palms necessary. By the way, if your babies actually grew in someone else's uterus, the more general answer, "All babies grow inside a woman in a special place called a uterus," would be peachy, too, and then just follow through with this way of phrasing things for the rest of the saga.

Age Five: How Did I Get Out of There?

Interestingly enough, it often takes children a whole year to ask the next logical question: "You're kidding, right? I was deep in your body? How on earth did I get out of there?" That's because at four they don't have the brainpower to step back and take in a process that big, and also, they just don't care to know about that yet. At five, though, they've moved on to a much more sophisticated understanding of time and place. The concepts of "before," "now," and "later" are now deeply embedded in their understanding of the world, and in their days, and they're not only interested in place but in things moving from one place to another. (Are you getting where I'm headed here?) Hence, their utter fascination with clocks, watches, and transportation vehicles of all kinds—and with labor and delivery. Movement through time and space, as in *transportation*—isn't that what labor is?

Once you have any kind of conversational history with your child about sexuality—in this case you both share the word "uterus"—you are in like Flynn. "Okay, remember last year when we said babies grow in their mom's body in her uterus? Well, right next to every uterus is another place called a vagina. It's a place made of two walls that touch each other but they can separate, too. When you were ready to be born, the uterus, which is like a muscle [you might want to take a side trip here to flex your biceps and demonstrate what muscles do], scrunched up and made itself really, really tight so it could push you out of its bottom part and then send you right through the vagina and out into the world." (And don't think you're off the hook if you had a C-section. You can also say, "And there's another way babies come out, too," and explain both at the same time.)

Age Six: But How'd I
Get in There in the First Place?

The six-year-old question is no simple query about concrete stuff like geography and transportation. It's about something much more mysterious, abstract, and invisible: the concept of *causation.* Newly able to grasp the logic and predictability of nature—as in, everything in nature has a cause, and every cause has an effect—sixes eventually get around to themselves: "I wonder what caused *me!*" They're also capable at this age of more sophisticated and convoluted mental gymnastics: "Let's review what I know so far. I'm *out here* now, but I used to be *in there*. I also know *how I got out of there*. But wait! Let me go back even farther in time and think about *how I got inside Mom's uterus in the first place*."

But there's more: a sudden and truly mind-blowing realization occurs to six-year-olds that brings it all together. Going back for a minute to five-year-olds to set the stage, if you happen to have one handy who already knows he grew in his mom's uterus, ask him, "Hey—where do you think you were *before* you were in Mom's uterus?" Since a five-year-old simply can't imagine a world without him in it, my bet is he'll merely offer up some location or another that makes sense to him at the moment: Heaven? Dad's uterus? Day care? The library? Sears? "If I haven't always been out here or in Mom's uterus," he'll reason, "I must have gotten there from someplace else!"

But a six-year-old eventually knows better. Much less egocentric than his younger self, he's willing to entertain that he's not at the center of the universe after all. His advancing computation skills will eventually seal the deal: "Let's see. Mom is thirty-two, and Grandma's sixty-one, and I'm six. Mom was twenty-six when I was born, and Grandma was twenty-nine when Mom was born, and . . . But wait! Mom wasn't alive when Grandma was little, so I wasn't alive when Mom was little! Good grief—that means I didn't always exist!"

So, truly, the six-year-old question isn't about sex at all. (By now this is no great surprise to you.) It's about the child's first awareness of the finite nature of her or his existence: Existentialism 101 for six-year-olds! As I said, mind-blowing. Doesn't it make you want to hug every six-year-old you know?

So how to explain this one? A good rule of thumb in talking to young children is to go from the general to the particular. "Here's a news flash for you, Malia: Mom and I made you all by ourselves!" Though this is a really neat idea, and Malia may think about and enjoy it for a while, as a cause-and-effect-oriented six-year-old, it's the "how" part that interests her most. "Yes, Dad, but *how* did you make me?"

"Well, Malia, *deep inside* Dad there was a tiny, tiny cell called a sperm. And *deep inside* Mom there was a tiny cell called an egg. And when they got together, that's how you got started. You started out as a tiny little speck, and just look at you now!"

Hmm, Malia is thinking. *Fascinating, but now I'm really curious.* (Of course she's more curious; Dad made sure to emphasize certain words to prompt her thinking—he wants her to keep asking questions because he wants to "get there first" and become her primary go-to person about sex, gender, and reproduction. (See Chapter 1.)

"But, Dad," Malia might ask, "how could something really little deep inside one person's body get together with something really little deep inside another person's body?" "What a great question, Malia. That's a hard design problem nature had to solve. Remember last year when we talked about vaginas, and the place between a woman's legs that babies come out of? Well, like all body openings things can go out *and* things can come in. So that the sperm and egg can come together, nature designed two female and male body parts—the vagina and the penis—to be able to fit together, sort of like puzzle pieces, so the sperm can come out of the penis and travel to the egg. By the way, when the vagina and the penis come together, that's called 'sexual intercourse.'" (Having a children's book with diagrams nearby would be great.)

Malia's likely response will probably shock you: "Oh." But that's exactly the point. She asked Dad a cause-and-effect question, and he gave her a beautiful cause-and-effect answer—just as he probably does at least five times a day, every day, with a curious six-year-old in the house. Please be aware, though, that Dad hasn't yet taught Malia *anything* about "sex," only about the juxtaposition of two particular body parts in the service of reproduction.

But suppose that isn't how Malia was conceived at all. Modern technology has created many new and different ways to conceive babies. What's more, families are formed in many different ways, too: single moms and single dads who make use of donated eggs or sperm, and maybe even surrogates; heterosexual and gay couples who have done the same; and all kinds of couples or individuals who have fertility issues.

If that's the case in your family, I would simply reverse course and start out with the sperm-and-egg part of the story: "Well, *all* human babies start out when two really tiny cells [it would be great to have a book handy about cells] called a sperm and an egg come together. One is from a woman and the other is from a man. There are a few different ways to put the two cells together, and here's the way it happened for you." Since young kids today go to school with children conceived in a variety of ways, many of whom are well educated and nonchalant about sharing how it happened for them, this might actually be a great way to start out with all children.

By the way, if part of you is still wondering whether this kind of information is *really* appropriate for young children to have, ask yourself the following: Is it okay to talk to four-year-olds about geography or five-year-olds about transportation, or six-year-olds about causation? Thinking of it that way puts it all in just the right perspective, I hope.

Folding in the Facts

Though my student didn't use the word "context" in her course comment, I think it's exactly what she meant to highlight. The ease of the conversations above, if you find them so, is totally attributable to the organic context that prompted them: the naturally occurring sequence of early childhood intellectual development. The topic wasn't sexual intercourse per se, but the ways in which children naturally need and want to think about it.

Context-making around sexuality is hard for American parents, since most of us learned about this subject haphazardly, from here, there, and everywhere, much like today's preteens and teens (except now "everywhere" literally is *everywhere*). If you didn't learn in ongoing, in-context ways yourself, it's hard to turn around as a parent and know how to create context around sexuality for your own kids. And for that you have come to the right book. Context is my strongest suit.

The easiest way to understand context-making is to think of it as a logical and comfortable "way in" to the discussions with your children you most want to have. Case in point: A slightly panicked mother of a ten-year-old asked me recently in a parenting class, "What do I do now? My son is having a puberty talk in school next month and I've never once talked to him about sex or babies in any way! How on earth could I bring it up now, like, totally out of the blue?" "Here's an idea," said one of the dads. "What's the chance you might someday soon walk by a pregnant woman?" "Oh yeah," she said. "My sister-in-law is pregnant and about to start showing. I could start there, couldn't I?"

Now, you know, if this were practically any other subject, she would have figured that out all by herself. As I said, when we don't learn in context, it's harder to create.

Some Great "Ways In"

Finding a comfortable way in to talking with your child about sexual topics is important not only for you, but for him, too. It takes away at least some of the awkwardness he may be feeling, and also gives him a means to prepare for, understand, and integrate what you are trying to say and why you are saying it. Learning for children is all about making connections. Here are twelve possible ways to create them, whether the topic at hand is factual or another kind of life lesson:

Developmental themes. So far we know that four-, five-, and six-year-olds, respectively, are wildly fascinated by geography, transportation, and causation, three concepts that just so happen to prime them beautifully for asking about their origins. But remember, these same three themes shape their thinking and curiosity about *everything* during those years. Perhaps your child never asked anything about her origins between the ages of four and six (and if she did, her questions may not have been in this particular order, or at these particular ages) but that's most likely because she just didn't get around to it; she was too busy thinking about geography, transportation, and causation in relation to *other* things. By the way, what prompts these questions is not some outside event, such as a pregnancy in the family or the birth of a sibling; the impetus comes from within, because the real subject is *me*. Reproduction is the answer, not the question.

As children and adolescents grow up, their questions about sexuality continue to mirror key developmental themes, creating constant openings if we're aware of them. As a teacher, for sure, child and adolescent development is my road map for knowing what to teach and when (and how). You probably spotted some great developmental ways in—even if you didn't label them as such—in the developmental profiles presented in Chapter 4. It's a good one to re-read as your kids grow.

Remember when? Having *any* type of conversational history about sexuality with your child creates a ready-made platform or context for conversations to come, as in the four-, five-, and six-year-old sequence above. This "remember when" approach can be used at any age to expand any topic:

✓ "Remember when we saw that TV show where the gay man was made to look as if he was more like a woman than a man, and I said that was a "stereotype"? See how that picture (or show, or movie) is doing the same thing?"

✓ "What does 'gay couple' mean? You know how Mom and Dad, and Aunt Dana and Uncle Elliott, and Arthur and Gloria loved each other in a special way and wanted to be together always and maybe start a family? Well, two men or two women can love each other in the same exact way. 'Gay' is a word for people who love people of their same gender."

✓ "What's rape? That's a hard one. Remember when we were saying that sexual experiences should always be something people freely choose to do? Well, sometimes one person forces another person to do something sexually they don't want to do, and that's called rape or sexual assault. Rape is a terrible thing and a very serious crime."

✓ "Hmm. The kids on the bus were joking about something called 'S and M'? That's like one of those sexual things we've been talking about that make people uncomfortable, so they laugh and make jokes. It's also something a lot of people think is bad or strange, because it refers to people who like to combine sexual experiences with giving or receiving pain, or pretending to do that."

By the way, even if you have no history talking to your child about sexuality, you really do: it's a history called "no history." You can always say, "Hey, there's a subject we never talked about before, and it's important that we do."

Preambles. If you've ever gone into your boss's office to ask for a raise, you probably practiced a preamble to the conversation: "I've been thinking about my performance in the Scott case, and it's clear to me that over the past year my work has reached a new level." Bringing up a sexual issue with your children can feel at least as intimidating as asking for a raise. A good preamble for an out-of-the-blue sit-down creates a verbal launchpad for whatever you want to say. Like these:

- ✓ "I know this is going to seem totally random (or awkward or out of the blue), and I wanted to say that upfront."
- ✓ "I want to bring up something that might be hard to talk about. It's really important. It might be slow going because I don't have a lot of practice."
- ✓ "I am really embarrassed about this subject, and maybe you are, too, but you know, we can probably talk and be embarrassed at the same time (and chew gum)."
- ✓ "We need to talk to you about something. We'll try very hard not to pry. We need to make sure you have some important information about safety."

Stage setting. If you know, for example, that your young child may be gearing up to ask how she got in or out of there, I suggest you make up a new family game beforehand called "let's name some body openings and tell what goes in and out of them, because that's what body openings are for," to set the stage for more easily and comfortably explaining sexual intercourse later on. If you have a middle school child who's squeamish about discussing "gross" topics, I'd try the "blow up" technique. Ask everyone in the family to share the very most gross and disgusting story they've ever heard in their life. (My personal favorite is about a woman who had a cockroach crawl up her nose. Really. I heard it on the radio.) After all that, vaginas are going to seem normal and even boring.

Or with a high school daughter or son, you might create a ritual, like Sunday breakfast out with Dad, for the stated purpose of catching up and talking to each other about life. You can eventually fold in sexuality as you wish, using other ways in to help you make the connection. Remember, your older children really do want to know what you think and value, but they may also feel some ambivalence. What often makes the difference is having a mutually comfortable and logical context to help set the stage. With any age child, shared time can become a gift you give each other. Find activities you can enjoy doing together, and take the time to interest and engage yourself in their passions, no matter what they happen to be. If you talk about things that have meaning to you both, eventually sexuality will fit right in.

Did you see/hear that? The bad news about the media is that it's everywhere. That's also the good news, since there are endless opportunities for teachable moments. Sometimes parents can overdo it: They try to talk to their kids about almost *everything* in front of them and end up driving themselves—and their kids—nuts. Not necessary! The most effective parents, I think, pick one or two TV shows (within reason) that their children want to see, especially programs that deal regularly with teenage issues, and carve out special times to watch with them together. Probably every issue you would like to talk to them about—factual, social, emotional, etc.—will show up in the story line in one form or another, in some ways you'll approve of and some ways you won't, and give you lots of opportunities to say what you think. Once they've heard you out, it means they've got your voice in their head and they've looked at the issue through your lens as a parent and caring adult. Then you're done! You can't make them think a certain way, of course, no matter how much you might like to. But you can make sure they think.

By the way, if your household doesn't own a TV, there are many great books your librarian can recommend for your kids on related topics that you can read together. Better yet, start a parent-child book club with like-minded parents.

Way backs. Isn't it so funny that when your kids are chatting up a storm with their buddies in the back of the car sometimes they forget you're there and don't think twice at all about what comes out of their mouths? If kids are young enough to be that naive, they probably won't mind you circling back at a later time: "Remember when you and Miriam and Daniel were talking about what Jessica said at lunch about Sara and Jack going into the back of the library to 'make out'? I'm glad I happened to overhear it. Let's talk about that!"

Zingers. Sometimes a zinger comes at you from one of your kids that leaves you literally speechless, if not hyperventilating. That's the nature of finding yourself in a context-free zone, a place where something feels so far out there's no way for your head to wrap around it. In other words, you can't for the life of you imagine a way in. Often zingers happen in front of strangers, "Mom, that metal box on the wall says T-A-M-P-O-N-S (or C-O-N-D-O-M-S).

What are T-A-M-P-O-N-S?" or totally out of the blue: "Daddy, what's oral sex?" Sometimes the worst zingers come at you through a third party: "Hello, this is the vice principal. We need you to come in to talk about some images on your child's social networking page that are causing quite a stir here at school."

Sometimes zingers are so off your radar they take your breath away: "Mom, I think I'm pregnant"; "Mom, I need birth control pills"; "Dad, I'm a lesbian"; "Mom and Dad, I feel like a boy inside, even though I'm a girl." Other times a zinger may be something you just happen to stumble upon, like an e-mail or text message laced with cruel comments (sent *to* your child or about to be sent *by* your child) or filled with vile or pornographic language. It's important to remember that what may seem like a lightning bolt to you probably isn't anything of the kind to your child. For her, it has a clear and very real context; she's just a curious girl who's fascinated by a new word on the thing on the wall in the ladies' room. Or a daughter or son who for days, maybe even years, has been rehearsing the announcement he or she just blurted out. Or a kid who thinks it's okay to do something if his friends are fine with it. Even if you're mortally embarrassed, or really angry, or disappointed, the important context to tap into is your child's.

Some zingers can rock your world to the core, but your child is still fundamentally the same child he or she was yesterday. You will adjust, and so will your children. Living through it together—and remembering that practically all parents face similar challenges eventually—will likely make all of you stronger. And it will make answering questions like "What's oral sex?" seem like a day off in the shade.

Do-overs. "Parenting is *always* a do-over" is one of my favorite things to say. It reminds us that we're human, after all, and that it's really okay to make mistakes with our children. I think of the word "mistake" quite literally as mis-take: If "Take One" didn't turn out to your satisfaction, or to your child's, there's always the next day, or month, or year to go back with a do-over. The one constant about our children is that they're almost always there tomorrow. What's more, kids love it when we own up to our mis-takes and aren't afraid to show our all too human side. Not uncommonly, it's they who end up comforting *us*: "That's okay, Mom. I know you were only trying to help me."

Often parents want to know how to go back and fix an untruthful answer they gave to dodge a subject they were afraid or too embarrassed to talk about with a child. Saying "I need to go back and correct a fact I gave you last month because I was trying to dodge a question that was really embarrassing for me" would do the trick. With a younger child, you can always say, "Last year when you were seven, and I told you moms and dads only have intercourse when they're making a baby, maybe like four times in their whole life, I left out a couple of details." They'll probably just be happy for the new information.

The rest of the body. One of the best ways to normalize information about the sexual and reproductive systems is to talk about them in the context of the whole body. The suggestion I made above about the "body-opening game" is a great example.

Here's another: My favorite way to talk to prepubescent children about puberty is to start out with a conversation about other body systems first, and then notice with them how the reproductive system works differently in fascinating ways from the rest. For one thing, each human being has only *half a system*! (Where would we be if we had bones on only one side of our body, or only the top half of our digestive system?) Not only that, but the half system each of us has only works on a part-time basis; it's not working yet when we're born, then it works for a few decades, and if you're a woman, it eventually stops working altogether. (What kind of trouble would we be in if our heart only beat on Thursdays?) Finally, the reproductive system is the only system in the body that individual people *never* have to use. (Good thing, since we only have half and it only works part-time.) Notice how the first point gives a logical opening for explaining sexual intercourse, the second for explaining puberty and menopause, and the third for letting kids know that over the years we adults will be back again and again for conversations about sexuality. Human beings, unlike animals driven by instinct, *make choices* about their sexual behavior; we can remind them, and it's up to us to make sure they know how to make wise ones.

Relate life to sex, and sex to life. In Chapter 1, I made the case that talking about sexuality with your kids is really talking with them about life. We teach our children life lessons all the time but often don't make direct connections from those lessons to this topic. So, if you're talking to your kids about bullying, for example, you can add something like, "There's another kind of bullying called 'sexual harassment,' when someone tries to make another person feel small and powerless by bringing unwanted attention to the sexual parts of their body. Do you ever see kids do that sort of thing?" Or you can go the other way instead: "That news story, about the woman who was being sexually harassed at work, reminds me of another one where kids were picking on a girl because she's an immigrant. Both stories are about bullying. Bullies almost always pick on something people can't change about themselves. They never play fair, and that's what makes them cowards."

Both/and. Sometimes we parents are full of "yes, buts" that keep us tied up in knots about talking to our children: "I don't mind telling my son about that, *but* he'll probably tell his little sister"; "I know she asked, *but* I really don't know how to explain it"; "I would tell him what I think about that, *but* I don't think he would listen." Once that little three-letter word creeps into the second half of a sentence, it discounts the first half and sabotages creative problem-solving: merely substituting the word "and" for "but" opens up all kinds of possibilities. You can still answer your child's question, *and* figure out a way to keep the information between the two of you. You can simply postpone answering a question ("Gee, I need some time to figure out how to explain that in a way you'll understand"), *and* then think it through or get help. And you can always start a conversation by saying, "I have something to say, *and* I'm afraid you won't hear me out." What a difference three letters can make.

How is an orgasm like a whistling teakettle? I use a lot of analogies in my teaching. It helps normalize the subject of sexuality for my students, by relating it to something they already think of as a comfortable, normal, and everyday topic. It also usually makes them laugh (or groan) and helps them think more clearly, as all good analogies do. Sometimes, for example, I give a quiz on reproductive parts called "Match the proper organ to the correspondingly shaped fruit, nut, or vegetable." (In the "apple doesn't fall far from the tree" department, my son delights us each week by likening the size of our daughter-in-love's pregnancy to—guess what—a particular fruit, nut, or vegetable.)

Like all analogies, these make what we can't see or understand directly more concrete and accessible. The only downside is that kids do complain I ruin certain foods for them forever. Did you know a placenta looks like a pizza on one side and a pancake on the other? (Sorry about that.)

My very favorite example is the uterus: Uteruses are shaped like small, upside-down pears, and the narrow part of the "pear" is called the cervix, which means neck in Latin. The outer, thicker part of the uterus (like the thick part of the pear that you eat) is made of muscle. At the bottom of the cervix is an opening (just like you could create in the top of a pear if you pulled out the stem) that lets sperm in and babies and periods out. The opening in the cervix is really tiny, which helps explains why labor is called "labor." It leads into a triangular slit-shaped area in the center of the uterus, which is where the lining grows and thickens (or where the pear's seeds are located). And as a seventh-grade student once pointed out, if a woman is wearing an IUD, the string for removing it, which comes down through the cervix, is analogous to the stem.

If you're still wondering how an orgasm is like a whistling teakettle, we'll get there, I promise.

Words, Words, Words

As most people know, the best time to begin teaching children a second language is when they are really young, because that's when the brain is at its most malleable. What people often don't realize is that American youngsters—mostly by osmosis and usually without a great deal of clarification from adults—are required to learn seven or eight different "sexual languages" all at once. With a few words for nearby organs and functions thrown in for good measure, here they are with some classic examples:

- *Proper:* vulva, penis, clitoris, labia, vagina, buttocks, urine, bowel movement
- *Babyish:* pookie, pee-pee, tush, tinkle, tee-tee, poop, wee-wee, go potty, ding-dong, ding-a-ling
- *Euphemistic:* going to the bathroom, fanny, down there, #1 (urinate), #2 (defecate), playing with yourself, the area covered by your bathing suit, privates, doing it, sleeping with, making love, thing, it

- ✓ *Descriptive slang:* balls, man in the boat or knob (clitoris), stiffy, woody, 'luter (for "saluter"—get it?), tool, rod, wiener, tubes tied (though that doesn't mean they can be untied)
- ✓ *Friendly slang:* Bob and the boys (penis and testicles), Ted and the twins (same), family jewels, honey pot, love pocket, rose petals, magic button, Johnson, Dick, Peter, Evelyn and Roberta (names for our breasts my girlfriends and I made up at Girl Scout camp one year), boobs, boobies, ta-tas, va-jayjay
- ✓ *Crude slang:* fuck, shit, cum, cock, jizz, piss, jerk off, jack off, blow job, eating out, eating at the Y, cornholing, mother fucking, screw, bang
- ✓ *Sexist/derogatory slang:* bitch, whore, pussy, cunt, fag, whipped, wimp, pussy, twat, snatch, tits, jugs, melons, rack
- ✓ *Technical/medical Latin- or Greek-based terms:* corpus lutem ("yellow body," referring to monthly changes on the surface of the ovary; there really is a "body" that turns yellow); bilateral partial salpingectomy (that's why people call it "tubes tied"); epididymis (my own personal favorite: "epi" in Greek means on and "didymis" in Latin means testicle, which tells you *exactly* where the epididymis sits)

What's a kid to do? Living in a context-free zone—with eight languages and dozens of words randomly bandied about (I actually once drove by graffiti stenciled onto a wall near Harvard that said "vas deferens")—how does a child make sense of it? Which language goes with which words? Where and when is it okay to use them, and not, and why? And by the way, what do all those words mean anyway? I liken it to the situation faced by an endearing twelve-year-old Russian immigrant I taught years ago at a local Jewish day school. He took one look at the vocabulary list I gave out to the class—sixty proper and technical terms—and panic splashed across his face. "I'm already having a really hard time learning to speak English and Hebrew," he told me. "Can you tell me, please, which words will be on the SAT, and is it okay if I just learn those?" "You're in luck," I told him, chuckling to myself. "I guarantee you *not one* of those words will be on the SAT."

This is what parents (and teachers, too) most need to recognize: all of these words are *just* words. We take the power out of them when we are willing to say them when our children say them to us, and we empower our children when we calmly explain how we feel about them, the rules for using them, and why the rules are important. In my classes, for instance, my students know they can say a slang word if they want to know what it means, or if it's the only word they know to express themselves, but they must always expressly ask the class's permission first, and then put "finger quotes" around the word when they say it; it's my way of teaching them that certain words aren't everywhere-anytime words—contrary to what they may see or hear around them every day. "Screw" is not like "foot," which you could probably say just about any time you felt like it.

Questions, Questions, Questions

It was legendary pediatrician and author T. Berry Brazelton who originally coined the phrase "anticipatory guidance." He used it to describe the reassuring process of educating parents about what to expect from children as they develop. So here's a handy and reassuring piece of anticipatory guidance for you to tuck away: your children could ask you a hundred different questions about sexuality, but they would really only be asking the same *eight root questions* over and over again. And I can even further reduce those eight to the magic number five, if you like, because each one of the eight is a reflection of children's fundamental needs, numbers one through five. Once this realization occurred to me as a teacher years ago, my shoulders dropped two inches permanently, because I knew, totally, what to expect on any given day.

Whenever your child asks you a question that throws you even a little, no matter what the question appears to be about on its face, ask yourself, "Which one of those eight root questions is this one about?" Knowing what you're listening for will help you avoid reading in, or projecting, what you think or presume or fear the question is about, so you can truly hear it for what it is. So here they are:

1. *What's true?* Now hear this: no matter what your mind or gut may tell you, the vast majority of questions that children and teenagers ask about sexuality are nothing more or less than *a simple request for the truth* about some new topic or another. And that piece of information, just because the topic is sexuality, is no more or less

inherently powerful, dangerous, or worrisome than any other kind of information. Once you see it that way, there's only one way to answer a "What's true?" question about sex—with the simple truth.

2. *How do people do that?* Questions about explicit sexual behaviors are also simple requests for factual information. So, just go back and re-read number one for guidance.

3. *Can you* please *help me figure this out?* This one's also basically a "What's true?" question. I hear it most frequently from frustrated middle school kids who are struggling with incomplete or partially inaccurate information. They're either trying to put two things together that don't seem to fit, sometimes very literally ("How do the penis and vagina fit together since the hole is so small?"), or they've got one piece of correct information combined with one that's incorrect. My all-time favorite example is, "What's 64?" because it's exactly half right and half wrong. (There was a rumor going around in the grade that "69" was really called 64.) These kids just need the truth, too, but they also need us to not chuckle or grin when we give it, since they don't know how adorable they are.

4. *How can I protect myself?* Here's the reason scare tactics don't work: teenagers just don't think about risky behaviors the same way as adults. When we hear bad news after bad news, our mind almost always eventually kicks in with some good news so we keep our balance. Not so with many teens. Too much scary information can cause them to feel overwhelmed, and they may react in the extreme, by going into complete denial ("that just *isn't* going to happen to me") or paranoia ("if that's going to happen, it *will* happen to me"). In neither case will they be able to process the information rationally.

So what I've learned to do is calibrate the facts I give, ever so carefully. I always give the honest and truthful bad news first—"Yes, gonorrhea can have scary consequences. Since girls usually don't have early symptoms, the infection can spread to the fallopian tubes and block them"—followed immediately by some good news: "There are ways to lower the chance of being infected in the first place, and also the germs can be picked up early on by scheduling routine exams." I know I've struck the right balance when the look on my students' faces says, "I've got it. This is scary and real stuff that I need to take seriously, but I know how to take care myself." I will admit, sheepishly, that if any of my students seem a little too relieved after I give out the good news, I usually sprinkle in a little bit more bad news to get the balance just right.

5. *Am I normal?* Kids don't usually ask these kinds of questions directly, so you've got to "lean in" sensitively to hear them. They might start out with the old standby, "I have a friend who . . . ," or seem a little—or a lot—tentative or nervous. They might have trouble making eye contact, or try hard not to sound too interested. (It's probably best for you to act that way, too. If you're drying the dishes, keep right on drying.) The right answer to this one, in every instance possible, is a resounding, "Yup. You're definitely normal all right." Kids worry about all kinds of things about their bodies, their thoughts, their behavior, and their fantasies, with very little comparative data to go on. They count on us to provide a big range of what's normal so they can fit themselves in.

6. *What should I do?* Younger kids especially ask us for advice all the time, and it's so very tempting, isn't it, to give it. Better, whenever possible, to show them a way to solve their own personal and social dilemmas. I often teach kids the acronym IDEAL I learned years ago: Identify the problem; Devise some alternatives; Evaluate each; Act on the one that seems best, or combine a few that will work together well; and Learn from the outcome. IDEAL is a little—okay, a lot— too hokey for older kids, but we can still walk them through the process by asking good questions. The hard part is stepping back and remembering who has the problem to solve: it's the child, not us. By the way, when it comes to sex questions, anxious parents (do you know one who isn't?) are prone to misread "What's true?" questions as "What should I do?" and fall into the trap of thinking, "If they want to know, they must be doing or about to do." Knowing is knowing, and doing is doing.

7. *What's right?* These questions are very different from the ones in category six. They're not about the practicalities of choosing a best alternative ("Who should I take to Prom?"), but determining *moral* rights and wrongs ("I asked Robby to the prom, but I really want to go with Hasim. How wrong would it be to disinvite Robby?") See Chapter 6, which is all about moral guidance.

8. *Will you pass my test?* Here's an adolescent law of nature: mixed messages from adults—US culture is a mixed-message factory, cranking them out incessantly, especially about sex and drugs—almost always invite testing behaviors. Kids want straight information from us about sexuality, and they'll often try to push our buttons to see if we mean what we say and say what we mean.

Testing questions can take many forms. Your son might ask a perfectly serious question with a too-playful glint in the eyes, slight curl of the lip, or joking-around tone of voice. He might lob the F-bomb or other such words just to see your reaction, or ask icky personal questions about your own sexual history. Since he's being manipulative, it will work best for you to be straightforward: "That seemed like a good and serious question, but I don't get why you're laughing or looking less than serious"; "When you use words like 'fuck' in that way, I wonder what your point is"; "That question about my sex life makes me extremely uncomfortable and put on the spot—it really crosses a line." Any one of these responses will earn you an "A" because you heard the *real* question beneath the surface and gave the best answer: "Yes, I will pass your test." With that out of the way, you can circle back and deal with the factual information he may be looking for: "Try your question again, but please ask it differently this time."

Be aware that sometimes these same behaviors may merely indicate embarrassment or your children's mixed feelings about the subject or about bringing it up. One way to tell the difference is by the way the behavior makes you feel. Testing questions usually make *us* feel really uncomfortable—that's the ultimate goal—whereas when kids are embarrassed or ambivalent it tends to make adults feel confused, frustrated, or annoyed. Your own feelings are often the best tool you have for making these fine distinctions.

Back to the Teakettle

You know the drill.

Repeat after me, five times: sex, oral sex, anal sex, sexual pleasure, S and M, "queef" (sound created by an air pocket in the vagina during intercourse), fart, tingly, pulsing, condom, nipples, orgasm, erection, ejaculation, clitoris, labia, stimulation, semen, erotic. Just words, right? You can't be a go-to person if you can't say them.

More context-making. Giving, hearing, and learning explicit sexual information is easiest when it's presented within a larger, nonsexual context. Here are some examples to help you gain more comfort and confidence in explaining what often feel like the trickiest of topics:

Sensory versus sexual: The body's sexual system, as I've said, is separate from the reproductive system, though the two overlap in important ways. It's part of the sensory portion of our nervous system, which enables us to feel, taste, smell, hear, and see. Like all other components of the sensory system, the sexual system produces very particular bodily sensations by *arousing* specific kinds of nerve endings, located in specific parts of the body. When there is no sound to hear, or sight to see, or fragrance to smell, our visual, auditory, and olfactory nerve endings are turned to the off or unaroused position. Add the proper stimulant, and—voila!—we suddenly see, hear, and smell, because the respective nerve endings are now turned on or aroused.

Sexual feelings work in exactly the same way. Most of the time we go about our business with our sexual nerve endings in the "off" position, but put us in any number of situations and—voila!—they literally turn on just like a lightbulb at the end of a switch. Gloriously pleasurable feelings emanate from our sexually wired nerves, sending waves of sensations—warm, tingly, excited, and otherwise hard to describe—to our sexual organs, and sometimes even our whole body. Our bodies are designed to be so sexually excitable that sensory input of any kind of can set off these feelings—sight, sound, taste, smell, and, of course, touch. Even ideas that just pop into our mind can do it. Sexual feelings just are; they're a normal, natural, and meant-to-be-enjoyed part of us. They feel good and they are good.

Sexual feelings can build and build in our bodies until they reach a peak of intensity called an orgasm. The whole process works, well, just like a whistling teakettle. When you first put a kettle on the stove, with the burner off, the molecules in the water just calmly sit around, waiting to gradually evaporate, as water molecules do. But if you turn on the flame and keep it on, they become more and more excited and start jumping around like crazy and hopping out of the water into the space above. Eventually the pressure inside the kettle builds to the extent that the steam forces its way up through the spout and out the kettle, and it has an orgasm. Once you take it away from the heat, the molecules settle down and go back to their previously unaroused state.

Parents, please don't say you'll never go into your kitchen (or make tea) again!

People enjoy many different ways of bringing their bodies together sexually. They hug, kiss, and touch and rub each other's bodies. They lie very close together and use their hands or their mouth, or both, to stimulate genitals or breasts to create pleasurable sexual feelings. Sometimes they bring their bodies together. When a penis and a vagina come together, that's called vaginal intercourse; when a penis and anus are joined, that's called anal intercourse; and when one person uses his or her mouth to stimulate a vulva or penis, that's called oral sex. Gay people, too, engage in all of these experiences, except the ones they're physically not capable of doing, because the two of them together don't have some of these parts.

Sometimes people use their hands, or maybe objects, to stimulate their own sexual parts to give themselves sexual feelings. That's called masturbation, or self-pleasuring. Our bodies are capable of all kinds of wonderful feelings, and we engage in many activities in life that give us pleasure, such as eating, sleeping, bathing, showering, swimming, diving, running, biking, exercising, getting a massage, and listening to music. And masturbating.

The magic of context, indeed. Just make sure your kids don't think that people automatically whistle when they have an orgasm (though some might).

Our "Gender Parts"

The confusion I hear from my students about their genital parts is exceeded only by what they don't understand about their "gender parts." What they reflect, as always, is how woefully undereducated Americans are about human sexuality, and how much misinformation they receive from peers and media. With so much sensationalism buzzing all around them today regarding gender and sexuality diversity, they've become increasingly attentive to these topics, and increasingly befuddled.

Gender is central to our identity, and is a part of children's fundamental makeup that grows and develops as they do. It has three separate components: biological gender, gender roles and expression, and gender identity. Understanding all three clearly, and especially how they're different, helps children better relate to themselves, their own development, and other people. Here's a fairly simple explanation of each that everyone should know.

Biological gender. I don't like to call us "opposite sexes" because we're not. Until each of us is about six weeks old in our mother's uterus, our genital tissue is exactly the same. We each have two separate masses of cells that aren't yet formed into specific parts (like lumps of genetic Play-Doh, as one of my students describes them), *and* we have tiny versions of *both* male and female internal reproductive parts. Isn't that interesting!

How we differ at this point is all in our genetics: males have an XY chromosomal pattern, and females, XX. Since Y is dominant genetically, embryos with XY become boys, and those with XX become girls. The Y chromosome is inactive until about forty-two days after conception, at which time it exerts its influence on one of the collection of cells I mentioned earlier to create testicles. They in turn manufacture the hormone testosterone. Testosterone travels to the second mass of cells and instructs it to become penis, foreskin, and scrotum, and also to the tiny internal reproductive organs where it instructs the male versions to continue to develop and the others to wither. In the absence of a Y chromosome, ovaries form, and there's no testosterone to "masculinize" the embryo anatomically. The same cell mass that becomes penis, foreskin, and scrotum in a boy, will become clitoris, inner labia, and outer labia in a girl (making us mirror images of one another, not opposites) and the tiny male reproductive organs will fade away.

With all these numerous and ultra-complex steps going on, there are bound to be variations, big and small. Some babies are born with external genitalia that don't match decidedly male or female patterns but are somewhere in between; some pop out with external female genitals, but testicles, not ovaries, inside; very rarely some, known as hermaphrodites, come equipped with both testicular and ovarian tissue inside. There are other variations as well. (For extra clarity: hermaphroditism is an extremely rare *form* of intersexuality; "intersexuality" and "hermaphroditism," therefore, are not interchangeable terms, though most adults and almost every child or teen I know misuses them in this way; some also think hermaphrodites are people with a full complement of both reproductive systems who could possibly impregnate themselves.) All of these individuals—more than 10 million, approximately, in the United States alone—are known as "intersexed." They are all part of nature's design. They push us to examine why we are so insistent that gender must be defined as such an either/or proposition.

Gender roles and gender expression. Gender roles are primarily learned. They consist of the social expectations society places on boys and girls and men and women because of their biological gender, which then become internalized as rules we adopt for ourselves. In American society, many traditional, long-standing gender roles have been under scrutiny for well more than a century, yet in many ways these expectations remain pervasive. They continue to prescribe how we are to live out our lives in minute detail—from the name we receive, to the colors, toys, and games we are supposed to like, to the clothes we are expected to wear, to the ways we talk, walk, communicate, and relate to other people.

Though we adopt and enact most gender roles pretty unconsciously, our gender expression—how we choose as individuals to put ourselves "out there" gender-wise, regardless of our biological gender—is much more conscious. Boys who choose, or are naturally inclined, to present themselves and act in the world in more traditionally feminine ways—or girls who do the opposite—are sometimes called "gender variant," "gender nonconforming," or "gender benders." They may refer to themselves as "transgender" or "genderqueer." By the way, lay terminology around gender and sexual diversity is evolving all the time, as our culture becomes more open to exploring these differences, so don't be surprised to see some of these terms used in a variety of ways. It can become pretty confusing, but I find that the best policy always is to refer to people in the way they personally prefer.

No doubt, biology plays a role in shaping gender role differences. If you're a man reading this book, for example, your brain was bathed in a significant amount of testosterone in utero, and mine wasn't. The field of brain science is learning more and more every year about gender-based brain differences, though this research is still essentially in its infancy. What we do know, without a shred of doubt, is that in countless (and mostly unconscious) ways, newborn baby girls and boys are held, spoken to, spoken about, played with, thought about, and encouraged differently, so that in the "nature-nurture" scheme of things, nurturing plays a huge role. Though many children from very young ages seem to gravitate toward traditional gender role behaviors and interests—and have parents who *swear* they didn't steer them that way at all—every one of them has been surrounded since birth by the gender-typed behavior of every single person they've ever encountered. There's no such thing as gender-neutral child rearing.

Gender identity. Gender identity is an entirely different matter. It cuts very deeply to *who we experience ourselves to be.* For most people, the gender they identify with psychologically perfectly matches their gender biologically; they feel a sense of total congruence in relation to their gender that they simply can take for granted. Other people, who self-describe as "transsexual," "transgender," or, increasingly today, as "trans," experience an emotional disconnect from their biological self; they feel the gender they are and the bodies they inhabit are a colossal mismatch. The discomfort with their bodies, and the huge strain and unhappiness created by having to live out their lives as a person they don't consider themselves to be, leads many with the funds to do so to undergo hormone treatments and eventually gender reassignment surgery. Other trans individuals, either because of financial reasons or simply because they are comfortable enough with their body as is, may undergo hormone treatments but never have surgery, or receive no treatments at all. In any case, it's not that transsexuals *want to be* the other gender; they know they already *are.* For those who undergo surgery, changing their bodies makes them feel right and whole and normal.

Sexual orientation. Sexual orientation is not a gender issue but a sexual one. Our sexual orientation—lesbian, gay, bisexual, or straight—is determined by the gender or genders we are sexually attracted to *in relation to our own*. It, too, is deep-rooted and not of our choosing. We either find people of the same or other gender, or both, sexually, affectionately, emotionally, and/or romantically attractive to us, or not. You may also hear two other terms pertaining to sexual orientation: "asexual," referring to individuals who experience no sexual attraction or desire for people of any gender, and "pansexual," describing individuals who find themselves attracted to people across the spectrum of gender and sexual variations. Sexual orientation for most people is fixed at a certain point in their development, but there are people whose natural orientation remains fluid and flexible throughout their lifetime. Young people should know that during early to mid-adolescence, feeling sexually attracted to or aroused by people of the same gender is not at all uncommon, and so are gay fantasies and same-sex experimentation. These experiences can be confusing for kids who, most of the time, self-identify as heterosexual. Most often they are not predictors of a gay sexual identity in late adolescence or adulthood.

Layers of Confusion

Americans very often conflate these four separate aspects of our sexual and gendered selves, despite the fact that they operate almost entirely independently. I hear kids—and adults—everywhere confuse the term "transsexual" (a gender identity issue) with "hermaphrodite" (a biological gender issue) and/or "transvestite" or cross-dresser (a gender role issue). What's more, many believe that all of these variations are somehow directly connected to being gay (a sexual orientation issue). It's important to help kids, and adults, get it all straight so they can better understand themselves and other people. Here's a way to explain the differences: People who are gay most often engage in the gender roles associated with their biological gender, just as people who are straight. A gay person's gender identity is almost always the same as his or her anatomy, and that anatomy is exactly what you would expect it to be.

One other source of misunderstanding is the idea that the dimensions of gender and sexuality manifest themselves in a binary fashion in human life: all people are either gay *or* straight, male *or* female, masculine *or* feminine, totally gender congruent *or* not. Not so at all!

As the paragraphs above reveal, each of these components expresses itself along a *continuum* of human experience. Most people do not fit neatly into binary categories or "boxes" in regard to sexuality and gender; humans are diverse in these ways, as in all ways. To acknowledge that labels of any kind are restrictive and misleading, many people now prefer the term "queer" as a way to describe themselves or others whose lives do not conform in one or more significant ways to society's binary expectations of sexuality and gender. Besides, they might argue, labels focus on how people are different, not how they're the same. *Everyone* has a sexual orientation and a gender identity, irrespective of what it happens to be, and that makes us all alike.

Finally, you've probably heard the acronym LGBTQ, which stands for Lesbian, Gay, Bisexual, Transgender, and Questioning, the last one for youth who are uncertain about their sexual orientation or gender identity and don't yet wish to label themselves. Sometimes there's an extra "Q" at the end for Queer.

There You Have It

As I'm always reminding teachers in training, there are many ways to do sexuality education well, but only a few ways to get it wrong. If you're a parent, not an educator, there's *always* a chance for a retake or do-over tomorrow, so relax and have fun with this amazing subject.

Here are some highlights from the chapter, to serve as a crib sheet of sorts.

- ✓ Most children have learned a great deal of sex-related information before they ever walk into a formal classroom setting; much of what they've learned is inaccurate and misleading.
- ✓ Between the ages of four and six, many young children spontaneously ask a predictable series of questions about their origins. These questions reflect universal developmental themes of the age and are not in reality about "sex."
- ✓ Inviting and answering these and other questions is the best way to establish yourself early on as a go-to person.
- ✓ Parents of children and adolescents often misinterpret their questions about sexuality, commonly because they project their own

anxieties and fears onto what they think their kids are asking (or doing).

- ✓ There are only eight root questions that children and adolescents ever ask about sexuality, and these are related to their five core nurturing needs. If you know what these eight categories are, you'll never be surprised.
- ✓ Children need to know as much about their gender parts as their genital parts.
- ✓ All words are just words. When adults refuse to say sexual terms, they diminish their ability to be go-to people.
- ✓ Embarrassment is just a feeling. The connection between sex and embarrassment is learned. It can be unlearned.
- ✓ Parents do not need to be experts on sexuality. They need to have a working knowledge of basic information and concepts.
- ✓ Context is every bit as important, or even more important, than content; context provides *meaning*.
- ✓ There are many logical and comfortable ways into conversations about sexuality.
- ✓ An orgasm is like a whistling teakettle.

6

Clarity About Values: Honing Your Message

Values and relationships are at the very heart of any meaningful dialogue about human sexuality. American popular culture, in glaring contrast, both glorifies and trivializes sex as a mere commodity, exchange, or transaction that happens most often between relative strangers. Just the titles of slick, star-studded films such as *No Strings Attached* and *Friends with Benefits*, released within weeks of each other in 2011, validate the idea of aimless nonrelational sex as the official, all-American standard. For parents who want their children to understand sexuality as meaningful and value-laden, that's an awful lot of stiff competition. This chapter aims to walk you through the process of becoming as clear and articulate as possible about the values you most want to impart to your children and teens, and to provide helpful ways into talking about them. You might need some patience in the earliest sections—it can be head-scratching stuff—but stick with me.

What Are Values?

I'm always struck by how imprecisely Americans define the word "values." A big part of the confusion, I think, stems from the multiple ways we use the word "values" in everyday speech. For example, we use it as a verb, as in, "I value my privacy, and my easy chair," and as the object of a verb, as in, "I value my privacy, and my easy chair; therefore, privacy and my easy chair are two of my values." And to make matters even more complicated, the concept of "privacy," for example, is a value in and of itself—one that some people value and some people don't. See what I mean?

Although it may seem as if I'm splitting hairs, there is a world of difference between those things in which we as individuals *place value* (our personal values) and those stand-alone principles or ideals that *in and of themselves are values.* Recognizing that distinction is absolutely crucial to communicating as clearly as possible about the whole topic of values, including, of course, sexual values. What follows is a quick primer on how to think and speak with this kind of clarity.

Personal Values

Personal values—which I call in my teaching "small-V values"—are those people, groups, places, things, ideas, memories, beliefs, ideals, experiences, activities, organizations, institutions, etc., in which a particular individual places worth. Personal values guide all of our everyday choices and help us divide up the pie chart of life in line with our limited time, energy, and resources. In fact, whenever we make decisions of any kind, we're weighing not so much our options but the relative merits of the values each one represents to us.

Everyone in the world has a one-of-a-kind—and ever-shifting—mix of personal values, different from those held by anyone alive or who has ever lived. Our values, in a sense, are "us." We arrive at them through a variety of life experiences, inborn preferences, and inherent capacities. Parents, relatives, upbringing, religion, laws, "society," friends, peers, role models, schooling, media, hundreds of other factors, and often just dumb luck and circumstances shape what we personally come to value.

Personal values can range literally from the sublime to the mundane—I personally value social justice, and also coffee ice cream with chocolate syrup—so the whole concept of personal values is somewhat nebulous. (All the more reason to define our terms carefully when we speak of them.) What's more, just because we *say* we value something, does that make it so? If we believe in a cause, for example, but never act on its behalf, can we legitimately call it a personal value? At the end of the day, it's our choices and actions that reveal what we truly hold dear.

Capital-V Values

Much of what we value in our lives is concrete and tangible. We can easily see, hear, and touch the people, places, things, possessions, activities, etc., that we cherish. As we grow up and develop the capacity to think abstractly, we begin to discover the huge, intangible world of ideas, ideals, and principles, and gradually begin to "own" and integrate many of these abstract concepts into our unique package of personal values.

Some abstract ideas are values in and of themselves. Embedded in these values are "shoulds" regarding human behavior—principles and ideals for determining whether a particular action is morally right or morally wrong. They provide ethical yardsticks for use in judging how human beings can best treat one another, other living things, and the natural and physical world. In my teaching I call these "capital-V values," "ethical values," or "core human values."

Whereas personal values are by definition *subjective*—what a person finds valuable is determined entirely from within—ethical values are *objective*, since, as I've said, they represent stand-alone principles that exist outside of us. To use a morbid example for the moment, when a person dies, her unique combination of personal values dies with her, because she is no longer around to value them, but ethical values will continue to exist in the realm of ideas out in the world.

The unfortunate phrase "situational ethics," popularized in the 1970s, has gradually eroded the public's grasp of the notion of "ethics," since many people eventually took it to mean that there are no definite yardsticks for determining right and wrong and that each situation must be judged entirely on its own *relative* merits. In fact, ethical values—such as equality, fairness, justice, sanctity of life, honesty, integrity, dignity, loyalty, mutuality, liberty, freedom, compassion, empathy, safety, privacy, respect, and responsibility—

are relative, but *only to one another*. (They're also internally consistent and interrelated—a real package deal). I may ethically take away the freedom of a person who is a danger to others, or tell a lie to save a life. But I can't pretend I'm making an ethical choice if I steal something from a store I really, really want but can't afford because my bank account is thin. One ethical value may trump another in a given situation (e.g., telling a lie to save a life), but personal values can't ethically do so.

So, Where Am I Headed with All of This?

A few years ago, a seasoned teacher in a training workshop I led made an observation that had heads nodding all around the room: "I just can't figure out what yardsticks kids are using today to make decisions about sex. Truthfully, I'm really not sure they're using any."

Though it's impossibly hard to make sweeping generalizations about "kids today" and what makes them tick—I know many, many teens who are exceptionally thoughtful and deliberate in making sexual decisions—I knew exactly what he was saying: Just how did sex become a literal no-brainer for a significant number of young people, devoid of any moral meaning or need for ethical consideration at all? The answers, I think, trace back to the seismic cultural changes that began in the 1960s, but once again, in much more subtle ways than may appear on the surface. Today's attitudes have as much to do with what *didn't* happen in the 1960s and 1970s as with what did.

In the evolution of American sexual values, "opportunity lost" is how I would characterize the latter third of the twentieth century. As I see it, the so-called sexual revolution was far less a revolution than a revolt; young Americans, especially, pushed and pushed hard against centuries-old sexual rules and values that no longer seemed to fit modern times. But most of the change that ensued was superficial and behavioral and *not* from the ground up, as befits a proper revolution. (The patriots didn't merely throw the redcoats out; they replaced colonial rule with a brand-new kind of governmental structure.) In the end, many of the older ways of thinking about sex and sexual morality had been chucked by a significant number of Americans, but the culture failed miserably to devise an alternative. The sophisticated moral reasoning that had once underpinned situational ethics[1]—involving the thoughtful application and balancing of capital-V values—evaporated like fine mist into the void, especially as marketers and popular media seized the opportunity to create a dumbed-down worldview of sex that would serve their commercial interests. (We're right back to the first sentence in this chapter, aren't we?)

In truth, I did witness a brief period of time in the mid-1960s when a real revolution might have taken hold. At the time a college student and young adult, I remember distinctly hearing the first sounds of change: "What does a piece of paper—as in, a marriage license—signify anyway? It's the commitment between two people to love and care about each other that really matters," or "What's important is that people take full responsibility for the consequences of their actions, physically, socially, and emotionally, and that they are honest with each other about their motives, desires, and expectations."

That shift in thinking signaled not a breakdown in moral values, as many claimed, but rather a shift in how one might choose to think about moral values. Whereas more traditional views of sexual morality are *rule-based*— "sexual intercourse belongs only in marriage"—this new alternative was instead *ethics-based*: "It's not marital status that determines the morality or immorality of sexual behaviors. The way to distinguish right from wrong sexual decisions is to measure them against core ethical values or yardsticks." Though a large cross section of Americans, then as now, support sexual values as seen through a more traditional or religious lens, adherents to this newer view argued for reliance on individual conscience and ethical reasoning— not prescribed religious, legal, or community standards—for evaluating sexual right and wrong.

That's hardly a "values-free" approach, and a very far cry from the "anything goes" tenor of the sexual "morality" popularized today. So, what happened? How did such large segments of the culture so quickly shift from a narrow, rule-based approach to sexual morality to one that's hardly about moral values at all?

Here's my take: Though a "rule-based" system for discerning right from wrong is fairly easy to understand and apply, a model that involves applying abstract principles requires learning how to think in a very particular and complex way that simply can't happen in the absence of deliberate adult mentoring. What didn't occur in the aftermath of the "revolution" was any kind of sustained attempt at mentoring the next generations of young people about sexual ethics. (What also didn't happen was the deliberate fleshing out of an ethics-based approach for general public consumption; the American Declaration of Independence would have proven inadequate without the seven years of painstaking work on the US Constitution that followed.)

Many teenagers I work with today easily articulate, and often subscribe to, the belief that sexual decisions have little to do with moral issues—that sex, essentially, is "amoral." They commonly frame it this way: "Sexual behavior is all up to the individuals involved. What is right and wrong is totally for them to decide. There *are* no objective standards, because all values are relative." Most also can readily identify traditional and religious-based rules pertaining to sexuality, and in fact they show genuine respect for peers and families who subscribe to these views. But for most of them, an understanding of sexual morality based on the ethical treatment of others is simply not in their awareness or their vocabulary. Though certainly they can name basic ethical values such as honesty and kindness, and easily explain why and how ethical values might be ultra important in *other* kinds of situations and relationships, when it comes to sexuality—beyond the issue of physical "protection"—they're most often at a loss to identify what else might be at stake. What they need, most of all, is serious and skillful mentoring by adults who can help connect the dots for them within an ethical frame.[2]

How Can Parents (and Schools) Help Connect the Dots?

In an earlier chapter, I wrote that when adults are clear about their own values it helps young children discover—in a world brimming with limitless options and possibilities—what is most important in life. Adolescents, too, benefit hugely from knowing their parents' specific views; it can provide grounding and guidance for some of the very first decisions they will make totally independently from us (which likely will include their sexual decisions, since we won't be there when they make them). It also bolsters them in the push/pull process of discovering their own identity. Sexuality is no exception; in fact, clarity from parents about sexuality is perhaps even more essential, given the constant noise and "buzz" about this subject from so many other competing influences. So, how do we get that clarity, and how can we make the case as effectively as possible that *our* values are well worth considering?

I always suggest that parents first think through some very pointed questions to begin the process of finding their own best answers and approaches. I've offered four important ones below, along with some of the ideas and experiences that have helped me shape my own answers as a teacher and a parent.

Question 1: What Does Sexuality Have to Do with Morality?

All moral questions deal fundamentally with our obligations to our fellow human beings and to ourselves. In planning a lesson last school year around the concept of sexual obligation for my high school classes, I thought to ask the following question: Suppose there are two people who hardly know each other who decide to engage in sexual intercourse, totally consensually and with appropriate kinds of physical protection. What are their personal obligations to each other?

The majority of the students, not terribly surprisingly, essentially answered, "Well, none." But—and this was the unusual part—when I went on to press them for an alternative point of view, if only for the sake of argument, they quickly became annoyed: "Hey, they're okay with it, they're each doing what they want to do, and that's that."

Well, that worked well, I said to myself, as I scanned my mind for another way to ask the question.

"Okay," I said, "let's change the scenario. Suppose there are two strangers who get on the train from Baltimore to New York City and end up sitting next to each other for two and a half hours. What are *their* obligations to each other?" The students, again, pretty much agreed: "None." But when I pressed them further on this one, with only a simple prompt or two, the answers just kept on coming: Well, you should say "excuse me" and be careful not to step on their foot if you get up to go to the bathroom; keep your elbows from crossing the center line between the seats, and your stuff away from their feet; if you talk on your cell, keep your voice low; if you've got a bad cold, be careful about spreading germs; maybe you could offer to throw out their trash when you get up to throw out yours; and try *really* hard not to burp or fart!

"Hmm," I said. "Here's what I think I hear you saying: There's a certain level of thoughtfulness and care people automatically owe a stranger they're sitting next to on a train, but not someone they get (at least partially) naked with and share intimate parts of their body. That's an interesting contrast! I wonder why the contradiction. What are your ideas?"

Then—and this is the really important part—I reminded myself to step back, be quiet, and let the students run the show. (As you probably know, too, this is not an easy thing to do, especially when kids say things that make you want to shake them or scream.)

Lots of good exchange followed as the students gradually reconsidered their hard and fast response to the first scenario and also contemplated why it might have occurred. Eventually I reminded them about the values discussions we'd had earlier in the week, and asked how these might connect to the scenario. They raised issues around respect, honesty, privacy, and kindness, and hashed out how, or if, they should be applied in this type of situation. They debated whether and when it was okay to treat another person as simply a means to an end, or to allow that kind of treatment of yourself, and then came up with sexual examples to test their ideas. (Girls giving oral sex to guys and expecting nothing in return created a lot of intense conversation regarding both the boy and the girl involved.) In the end, most were left challenging their original assumptions—my most important job!—in this case, about what any two people sharing a sexual experience might owe each other simply because they are fellow human beings. One girl, contemplating her own originally blasé response, summed up what she thought was a major point: "We seem to forget that *people* have sex, not body parts."

Another crisp realization for some was that, despite the "shoulds" we'd just been discussing, as a practical matter no one really can count on anything from a person you barely know, nor they from you; several found that a sad and odd context for a sexual experience. At some point I added that try as people might to compartmentalize their physical and emotional selves, we truly do bring *all* of ourselves with us wherever we go, and sex is no different. That's why "no strings attached" sexual experiences can create surprising or unexpected social and emotional vulnerabilities, I said, and also why many people insist on developing a significant level of trust in a relationship before turning their body over to another person.

Once youngsters enter adolescence, they appreciate it most when adults engage *with them* in this kind of four-step process: (1) holding up a mirror to life in a nonjudgmental but interesting way; (2) asking a thoughtful question; (3) really listening; (4) eventually adding your own opinions and your adult perspective. When we "trust the process," as a counselor I know always says, we often get a whole lot further than when we try to tell kids what to think or do. We also create the kind of trust that makes adolescents want to hear what we have to say, too.

In as many compelling ways as I can, I work especially hard to "hold up the mirror" to American popular culture, to help take kids out of the water they swim in 24/7/365 and don't even realize is there. It's one of my best tools for combating the media-created disconnect between sex and people's basic humanity. (Once that connection is gone, why *wouldn't* kids think that sex is fundamentally amoral?) And it almost always provides opportunities, as in the example above, to use lessons about life—in the conversation described above, an ordinary train ride—to bring clarity to sex.

I also like to connect the dots for my students—starting in late elementary school—about the potential power that any kind of sexual experience can create in people's lives. To demonstrate this point to yourself, think back a moment to the very first "real" kiss you ever experienced: How old were you? What were the exact circumstances? What were your thoughts and feelings at the time? How much do you remember? Did it change you? How?

My personal answers, in case you're at all interested: I was thirteen, it was April, and I was riding in the backseat of a car with Mark B. It was a Saturday night, right around 11, and just before he kissed me I was thinking about having to get up early the next morning for religious school. I was wearing a plaid dress, he a jacket, shirt, and dark tie. His prematurely graying father—I know this because I had my eyes fixated on the back of his head, petrified he would turn around and catch us—was driving us just past the 3900 block of Garrison Boulevard in Baltimore City, not far from Liberty Heights (of movie director Barry Levinson fame).

I felt, approximately in this order: surprised and slightly embarrassed; worried about my breath; insecure that I was probably doing it wrong; very disappointed in the texture of his lips; excited and grown-up and happy to be more like my friends; good about myself, because maybe Mark really liked me; awfully confused because it wasn't at all what I expected; and guilty because I knew in that instant I was going to "break up" with him. (This was truly a nine-second relationship; I'd secretly had a crush on Mark, well, forever, but after those nine seconds I knew I would have to move on with my life.)

That kiss totally changed my early teenage social world, and some kisses in history have changed *the* world. Imagine. "Just" a kiss!

By the way, if you, too, remember a "first" in some detail, exactly what else do you remember quite as vividly from that particular year of your life? (Me? Nothing!) And be sure to take note, of course, that these early experiences are just as powerful for kids today as for generations past. They can make for great—and fun—discussions with young teens, and they allow you to make a point of saying, "If that's how powerful a kiss can be, imagine the intensity of a much more physically intimate sexual experience."

And if you really want to talk to your kids about sex and power, ask them to consider the fact that vaginal intercourse, without a doubt, is the most fundamentally powerful behavior on the face of the planet: Within the space of ten seconds—because that's how long ejaculation takes—it has the power to accomplish not one but three of the most powerful things there are, all at the same time: (1) create new life; (2) potentially take life away; and (3) change any number of people's lives *forever.* In my book, that kind of power creates a huge obligation to self and others, and commands utmost respect for the act of sexual intercourse itself. It's a fact of life I start talking to my students about in the fourth grade.

I think we have to be direct and honest with teenagers of all ages that two people can and do meet, enjoy a very physically satisfying sexual experience together, and go their separate ways. At the same time, we also have to be prepared to explain how that kind of encounter is potentially light years away from an experience between two people who really know and feel emotionally close to each other. I liken it to sitting at a table enjoying a scrumptious five-course gourmet meal all alone, compared to sharing the same luscious experience with someone you truly care about and who cares about you, while laughing, and talking, and sharing endearments. One of my biggest worries is that too many kids won't know their real options if we can't or don't explain them, and will cheat themselves out of understanding, wanting, and knowing how to create truly intimate sexual experiences.

Question 2: What Values Do You Want Your Children to Bring to Any and All of Their Sexual Experiences?

Suppose I gave you a magic three-by-five-inch file card. It's magic because if you fasten it to the surface of your child's most frequently used mirror, it will immediately become embedded inside and no one will be able to remove it until your child's twenty-first birthday. If the mirror breaks, or if you move away, or if your child leaves to go to school, it will magically reappear in his or her *new* most frequently used mirror. There will be no escape!

On the card you can write up to eight values you hope for, want, and expect your children to bring to *any and all* sexual experiences in her or his life, including first kisses.

What would you put on the card?

It's fun and really revealing to ask a roomful of parents to write down their answers in small groups and then share them with everyone. There are usually a number of "a-has!"—for everyone. The first is that practically everyone in the room has produced virtually the same list. (We tend to think Americans are all over the map in terms of sexual values, right? Not so.) What a huge and fertile ground of common values we could choose to stand on for all of our kids' sake in a world where outside of family, school (maybe), and clergy, they get nothing but mush. And another quiet bombshell: the list includes the *exact same values* parents are working hard to teach their children about everything else in their lives, but maybe haven't thought to connect in ongoing and direct ways to sexuality.

In other words, the values on the list are all some combination of values with a capital V: honesty, trust, respect, responsibility, integrity, freedom (to make your own choices without pressure), fairness, loyalty, dignity, caring, compassion, empathy, safety, and privacy. As soon as they start tumbling out, I feel as if the "opportunity lost" of the mid-1960s and 1970s is found: parents are learning to think about sexual choices through the same ethical lens that applies to *all* human behaviors involving treatment of self and others.

These are some of my very best moments. It's impossible to overstate the importance of parents making those connections for themselves, and for their children. There's no more powerful way to counter the effects of America's culture of disrespect around sex, and gender as well, because it keeps the focus on the human beings attached to the physical parts. In a society that obsesses over the physical, the questions we most often ask about teenage sex center on what teens are doing, not the context in which they are doing it. Unless and until we attend to the humanity of sexual experiences, we'll continue to reinforce in our minds and theirs that sex is about body parts, not people.

Question 3: When It Comes to Sex, What Kind of Moral Thinker Are You: Ethics- or Rule-Based?

I've never met a parent who wouldn't or couldn't sign on to capital-V values, or who didn't hope their children would, too. (Living by them all the time is another story altogether; who does?) For many parents, knowing their children are striving to make caring, respectful, and responsible choices around sexual behavior is sufficient from a moral point of view. Others, who also value these ideals, may believe they are morally necessary, but not always morally sufficient. Whether because of family traditions, cultural attitudes, or religious beliefs, these parents are deeply concerned not only with *the way* their children make sexual decisions, but also *the specific decisions* they choose to make.

Many parents participate in religious traditions that are vitally important to them and their immediate and extended families. To them, defining morality solely in terms of ethical obligation in the mortal world misses the point entirely: one's first and most important obligation is to God and God's laws; ethical codes of conduct follow from that. The Ten Commandments, contained in the Old Testament and common to Judaism, Christianity, and to a large extent Islam, make clear the primacy of God and God's laws. Though the last six commandments underscore ethical values, such as respect, the sanctity of life, fidelity, and honesty, the first four lay out the requirements for one's relationship with God. Moreover, there are also parents who draw enormous strength and guidance from decades– if not centuries–old family and cultural norms and traditions, many of them entwined with cherished religious values as well.

Parents whose sexual values are primarily ethics-based face a challenging task: teaching young people how to think about sexual choices is a more complicated and nuanced task than suggesting (or dictating) what those choices should be. An ethics-based view centers on the *how and why* of human behavior, not the particular sexual behavior itself. That's why ongoing mentoring—modeling, naming, highlighting, reinforcing, and helping children apply ethical values to sexual situations, just as they might in all other areas of life—is so very important. The lessons these parents teach will emphasize values such as privacy and respect (it's wrong to blab about what you and another person have done sexually, and even worse to boast about it); honesty and empathy (it's wrong to tell people you like or love them so they'll agree to do what you want sexually); and the balance of freedom and responsibility (sexual experiences are potentially very positive and fulfilling, and also powerful physically and emotionally; great care must be taken).

Many other parents come from a perspective that is more rule-based or "act-centered." For example, many religious sects strictly prohibit birth control, abortion, premarital intercourse, masturbation, homosexual conduct, or other specific sexual acts; many families and cultures embrace similar rules as part of long-standing traditions. For these parents, there are certain decisions where ethical values—except for loyalty to God—become entirely secondary, if not irrelevant; if you consider abortion or premarital intercourse to be absolutely wrong, for example, no decision-making process, no matter how thoughtful and ethically based, will ever make it right. Parents who want their children to equally cherish both ethical values and strict religious doctrine must learn to walk a proverbial fine line—especially with adolescent children, who typically have built-in radar for what strikes them as contradictory or hypocritical. It's good to acknowledge the incongruity up front, and it's a good time to make use of a "both/and" approach: two contradictory ideas can coexist in the world, one based on the laws of people, and the other the laws of God.

Some of my students, quite honestly, are prone to discount religious guidance about sexuality. They are quick to assume that religion is mostly about rules that are "against sex" or that just tell you what you can't or shouldn't do. If faith-based beliefs are important to you, making sure you—*and* your children's religious educators—frame views on sexuality in a fundamentally positive light is really important. In my case, as a Conservative Jew,[3] that's easy.

The message to young people, unequivocally, is that sex is good and a gift from God; it has the power to give unspeakable pleasure, to create a deep and lasting bond between two people, and to give new life. Because of its extraordinary goodness and power, it is not to be treated as ordinary, but elevated as separate and holy, just as the Sabbath and all things connected to God. Sex between a committed couple is considered a "good deed," except on Shabbat, when it counts as two good deeds!

In extreme cases, parents reach the conclusion they must choose between their deeply held traditional or religious beliefs and their teenage or adult children who take another path. These situations are among the most gut-wrenching and hurtful imaginable and usually create life-long scars, especially for youth, who desperately need to count on their parents' unconditional love. It is always best to find a way to avoid this kind of breach. There is great concern, especially, about young people who identify as lesbian, gay, bisexual, or transgender, since the rejection they may experience from parents and others cuts directly to the core of who they experience themselves to be. In recent years, a spate of high-profile suicides among this population of kids—virtually all of whom experienced constant condemnation from family or peers—have made all too vivid the tragic consequences for kids who face inescapable hatred, rejection, and the overwhelming hopelessness they can create. What's more, in recent years teens and children have begun "coming out" to themselves and others at significantly younger ages. All parents are wise to educate themselves about these issues for the sake of all of our children.

The "gut" factor. When it comes to sensitive topics, such as sexuality, it may be hard at times to put your finger on exactly why something seems right or wrong to you; you just sort of feel it in your gut. For one reason, there are attitudes toward sexuality we learn as young children, not in a conscious way but on an emotional and experiential level, that are hard for us to access decades later through our intellect. Often we're not aware of them until an experience or event brings them to the surface.

Also, for many people there's an "ick" or "yuck" or "disgust" factor connected with certain sexual practices. Bestiality and necrophilia (sex with animals and dead bodies, respectively) accomplish this for most people! Pornography, fetishes, sadomasochism, transvestism (needing to wear "opposite"-sex clothing or underwear to achieve sexual arousal) can arouse viscerally negative judgments as well. Other folks feel disgusted by behaviors such as anal sex, oral sex, or self-pleasuring. Truthfully, it's a good exercise to try to sort out your feelings around these kinds of behaviors; they can help sharpen your skills at separating ethical, rule-based, and strictly gut-based reactions and attitudes. That will be useful for your children, who very well may hear about such things and come to you for information or your opinions.

By the way, when they do come talk to you about these kinds of topics, it's a terrific sign that you are definitely their *major* go-to person. Enjoy the moment (even if the topic is necrophilia!).

One final thought: out of our love and the overwhelming desire to protect them and because, to a degree, we can't help see them as an extension of our own ego, we parents probably "think with our gut" most of the time about our kids. This is not a bad thing. Coming to terms with our children's overt sexuality, though, can be terribly complex, and our gut reactions can become overwhelming. For example, parents who find out that their children are involved in a sexual relationship often find it hard to get out of their gut and up to their head so they can think rationally. In such situations, it's time for an honest and deliberate "gut check." It really helps to put your reactions down on paper—*before* you talk to your son or daughter, if that's your plan— then check off the ones that come from your own "stuff" and deal with them separately. You'll keep your focus more easily on the issues that truly revolve around your kids and *their* needs.

Question 4: What Are Your Personal Beliefs and Values Connected to Sexuality?

As a parent, what's most important is taking stock of your views, including where they come from and why they're important to you. Identifying which are based on ethical considerations, and which are grounded in rules and values you've chosen to honor out of devout faith or tradition, helps you hone the messages you most want to give your kids. Notice especially if your head, your heart, and your gut don't seem to be aligned, and think that through, too. Own all of it, and explain it to your kids. And then sit back and listen.

Here are a few questions to help guide your thinking, clarify your values, and put them into words your children can understand and make use of. Pick the ones you find most helpful. Then think, write, and/or talk them through with someone who's a good listener and sounding board.

- To what extent were your parents' views about sexual behavior rule-based? Ethics-based? Gut-based? How do you know?
- Were there sexual experiences you engaged in as a teen that your parents would have approved of? Been proud of? Disapproved of? On what basis?
- If your children were to ask, how would you define "responsible sexual behavior" beyond the issue of physical protection?
- What is your moral take on sexual behaviors such as anal sex or oral sex? Are there "gut" reactions about the specific behaviors that factor in?
- At what point along the continuum of sexual behaviors—from hand-holding to various forms of intercourse—do moral, ethical, or religious standards apply? Why do you choose that point?
- In your mind, what are acceptable reasons or motivations—and not—for teens saying "yes" to a sexual experience (along the continuum)?
- What are your views on abortion? Gay marriage? Gay rights? Are your ideas based on your gut, traditional or religious teaching, and/or ethical considerations?
- If religious faith is important to you, do you ever disagree with its tenets or practices from an ethical point of view? If so, how do you wrestle with those discrepancies in your day-to-day decisions or in your mind? Do any of them relate to sexuality? How would you explain your struggle to your children?
- What will or should be your reaction if your child violates one of your most cherished personal/traditional/religious rules or values? Would it make a difference to you if his or her decision-making *process* was grounded in ethical values you admire?
- Rethink the above questions, if you haven't already, in regard to children of both genders, and/or as the parent of a gay, lesbian, bisexual, or transgendered child. Are there differences?
- Share these questions and your answers with your partner, spouse, or co-parent, and ask him or her to think and share, too. What are the areas of agreement and disagreement? As parents, how can you best handle important differences between you? Which of the other

person's views are rule-based, ethics-based, or gut-based? How do they compare to yours in that way?

What About Abstinence?

"Abstinence" is a word I always use carefully and purposefully. Without context it's an empty concept: What does it really mean, and what kind of guidance does it really provide? When I hear other people use the word casually, I always want to ask a whole bunch of questions: Abstinence from what behaviors? With whom? For what reason? Under what circumstances? For how long? Unless we build in concrete guidelines (i.e., specifically what, when, who, and why) to our messages about abstinence, we may feel we're being responsible adults by talking about it, but in the end, for our kids, it might not be terribly useful. They need well-defined handrails to lean on.

Remember, too, that in a culture where 99 percent of the time the word "sex" is meant and taken to mean "sexual intercourse," when adults say things like "abstain from sex" without specifying what kind or kinds of sex they do or don't mean, young people may reach conclusions we don't intend and that might actually be dangerous. Some teens, for example, will say and believe they are abstinent—and safe from sexually transmitted infections, or STIs—because they've not engaged in vaginal intercourse, even though they have engaged in oral and/or anal sex. All three of these sexual behaviors, of course, can expose partners to STI germs. In addition, from a values perspective—particularly ethical values—if we say "sex" and really mean "intercourse," we give a powerful message by default: "When it comes to other sexual behaviors, ethical values and thoughtful decision-making about abstaining or engaging need not apply." In reality, of course, issues concerned with "treatment of self and others" are embedded potentially in any sexual experience; that's a message I think we want our kids to get, deeply, before they engage in any of them. It's also the best buffer we can create against the influences in their lives that depict sex in any form as an amoral proposition.

It's helpful to be clear—and to make clear to your kids—specifically where advice about abstinence is coming from, since there are multiple possibilities. Your concern may be *developmental* and/or *health related,* because you know certain sexual behaviors are beyond your child's level of maturity or carry too much physical, social, or emotional risk. It may be *ethical,* for example, because you question the motivation behind your son's or daughter's sexual choices. It could be *relational*; you might be convinced that sexual involvement is premature for your child given the nature of the relationship in which she or he is involved. Or it could be *religious,* if a behavior is not in line with your cherished beliefs or values.

In this last example, if chastity and not abstinence is the real issue at stake for you, that might be a compelling distinction to draw for your child. Whereas abstinence is a behavioral choice that people make under a variety of circumstances and for a great variety of reasons, being "chaste" is more powerfully described and understood as a spiritual state of being. If that's a cherished value for you, stating why, from your heart, can give your message additional meaning and "punch."

Finally, I always feel conflicted when I see "abstinence" on a list of birth control methods. For sure, people at times choose to abstain from sexual intercourse for fear of pregnancy (or disease). But abstinence is an ongoing *life choice,* not a birth control choice. People choose to take a pass on—or take part in—all kinds of sexual experiences for all kinds of reasons. One study[4] revealed 237 reasons why women say yes! The researchers didn't ask why women say no, but that list for sure would be just as long. What our children need to know is how to decide which reasons are the best and right ones. The "Okay/Not Okay/Not Sure" exercises that I describe at the end of the chapter is an interesting and engaging way to ask kids, especially middle schoolers, to evaluate possible reasons for saying yes or no to *any* sexual experience—from kissing to oral sex to intercourse. Be sure to make the point that *any* reason for saying no to *any* sexual experience must be respected by the other person. In fact, no one is obliged even to give a reason: no means no, no matter.

Avoiding Mixed Messages

Very often parents tell me they are very worried about giving their children mixed messages about sex. How can you avoid it, they say, if you prefer your child not participate for any number of reasons, but you feel you must talk to them anyway about "protection"? (First, of course, I ask them to tell me what kind of "sex" they are referring to and what they mean by "protection.")

What it usually boils down to is something like this: How can you be credible if your message is, "Don't do that or I'll kill you, but if you do, use a condom"?

No wonder they're perplexed: they are trying to make a peanut butter and jelly sandwich without the bread! When advice feels mixed, or really gooey, to continue my analogy, it's a sign you're probably not stepping far enough back to see what the individual messages have *in common*. In this case, it's all about protection, and here's the "bread": "We love you and *always* want you to be safe. Our very best advice is to postpone that behavior. If it ends up that you make another choice, here's information you'll need to have." The *real* mixed messages about sex come from a popular culture that beams the opposite of protection at our kids all the time.

Nurturing Your Children's and Teens' Ethical Compass

I know a couple who are raising their five children very deliberately with core ethical values as an everyday part of their family life. They long ago decided the right way to fortify their children against "junk" culture was to treat it like junk food. They don't hide it, but they don't often make it available either, and they make sure to feed the kids healthy alternatives that taste good and are nutritious, too. Their children could talk intelligently about food ingredients and analyze the nutrition labels on packages by the time they could read. Soon they were helping to select products in the grocery store by comparing the labels, and gradually they all learned to plan and prepare healthy meals, eventually entirely on their own.

In a parallel way, the parents helped each child build an ethical vocabulary, introducing a new word—fairness, kindness, honesty, loyalty, equity, safety, respect, compassion, responsibility, empathy—whenever it was a natural fit, even if it was too big a concept at that moment for the child to grasp. By deliberately pairing each word over time with clear, concrete examples—"we take turns in this game because that's what's fair"; "to be fair, everybody will get exactly five pretzels"; "hold on, let's show your brother some empathy and find out what made him angry"—the words became part of a working vocabulary for ethical thinking. Even the youngest, a pair of eight-year-old twins, can name them, extract them from all kinds of situations—"the girl in the story is kind but not honest"—and apply them at will to their own behavior or others'; these are not simply words.

Conversation with their middle school–and high school–age kids often revolves around more abstract ethical values—equality, social justice, integrity, fidelity, human dignity, and the balance of freedom and responsibility—in regard to both national and international events and also interpersonal relationships and decision-making, with issues around sexuality and gender thrown naturally into the mix. (The daily news is filled with stories relating to sexuality and gender in important ways.) And everyone in the family knows that these are *human* values, applying equally to boys and girls and men and women, even if other influences around them (including "junk" culture) don't seem to agree.

These parents make sure, as often as they can, to *name and apply the values they want their children to value.* They're convinced that's every bit as important to a good and healthy life (including a happy, healthy sexual life) as eating protein and avoiding saturated fat.

Gender, Sex, and Values

Among the strongest influences on young people's sexual attitudes and decisions—and often the most negative—are cultural perceptions and representations of gender. Underneath our supposedly "postmodern" and liberated society lurk powerful, antiquated stereotypes of men and women and how they are supposed to relate to one another. And with the exposure of younger and younger kids to adult-themed material in movies, song lyrics, and video games and on TV and the Internet, the "role models" today who teach them the most about relationships between the genders are likely to be actors, celebrities, entertainers, fashion models, action figures, and even cartoon characters. That's a lot for parents to pay attention to and help their children unpack. Here are some important issues to think about addressing.

Liberation or Exploitation?

One source of concern—and consternation—for many parents, and maybe you as well, is the sexualized way that many teens and even younger girls now choose to present themselves to the world. What seems to bother many parents the most is not simply the overt "sexiness" of the look, but rather what they perceive as girls' utter cluelessness and naïveté—particularly when they insist, as some girls do, that being free to show off your sexuality is a sign of liberation from outdated stereotypes and other repressive influences. "Don't they realize that they are only inviting their own objectification?" a typical mom asked me recently. "What's happened to make our girls so blind?" she continued. "Weren't the 1970s, like, more than thirty years ago?"

What Ever Happened to "Feminism"?

Answering that question would take more than a whole shelf of books by a bevy of social historians. But I can definitely report that over the years I've known fewer and fewer young women in high school who will own the word "feminist." Many girls actually know very little, if anything, about the history of the women's movement, and those who do very often don't want to associate themselves with the negative and off-putting stereotypes (bra-burners, men-haters, "dykes," etc.) they've heard used to describe women from that period. I've known girls, too, who are very aware and sensitive to gender issues, but who shun the label because they've witnessed firsthand the ridicule sometimes directed at girls who speak up about gender inequities they see or experience. Many moms, too, share bitter frustrations with me about trying to "raise consciousness" at home with daughters and sons, only to be told they're just "oversensitive" and annoying.

In the minds of many other girls and young women, the battle for gender equality has been won; they simply consider themselves already "equal" to their male counterparts. Especially for those with the tools to fund education after high school, the future does indeed seem bright. Since the passage in 1973 of Title IX, the federal statute prohibiting gender discrimination in education, years of hard and focused work has clearly paid off, with women now plainly outnumbering men in many colleges and professional schools. (What girls don't often foresee are the inequities they may yet confront; a year out of college, according to data from as late as 2008, they'll be making 80 percent of what men in comparable positions earn, and after ten years, only 69 percent.) Some experts even suggest that girls, in fact, are "more equal" today and that it's time to put the focus on boys who are lagging. Though I don't agree at all that this is a zero-sum proposition—that helping girls ever means taking away something from boys, or vice versa—for sure, many goals of the movement are being realized for an increasing number of girls and young women every day.

But What About Sex? Is That "More Equal," Too?

I wish I believed that were true. I fear that what many girls view as a sexually leveled playing field may be an illusion. It's curious, isn't it, that one of the longest-standing and most blatant forms of gender inequity remains, even today, fundamentally unchallenged: the sexual double standard. Though most girls I know are savvy enough to spot and object to favoritism toward boys in classrooms or sports in a heartbeat, the fact that the sexual double standard is rigged, and not in their favor, is pretty much accepted as "just the way it is." It's minimized further by what Susan Douglas, professor of communication at the University of Michigan, describes as today's "enlightened sexism."[5] Media and pop culture, she argues, continually fuel fantasies that feminism, and its pint-size version, "girl power," have been such an unqualified success that it's now right and okay to resurrect—and even celebrate or flaunt—sexist stereotypes that no longer matter. Marketers spend billions, she contends, convincing women and girls that *sexual power*—to be maximized, of course, by the products they sell—and *real power* are one and the same.

Some years ago I went into the county clerk's office at my local courthouse to file a legal paper. Behind the counter was a woman wearing a very low-cut, tight-fitting top. Her breasts caught my attention the second I walked in, and frankly, I could not get them out of my mind, or the corner of my eye, even as we were speaking. The next week I went in again, only to find a (fully clothed) male clerk instead. As I looked into his face and listened to him, undistracted, I took in his intelligence, his earnestness, and his smile. He was a whole person to me, not a talking head attached to a sexualized body. It was a fascinating juxtaposition, and it taught me a great deal. I thought of the two of them again when I came across Douglas's work, and how strikingly the woman's overt sexuality, in this situation, worked directly against the *real power* she held just by being herself.

Women have always used their sexuality and their bodies to garner attention, particularly from men who could offer them access to the power and money societies denied them directly. The important question to ask, I suggest to my teenage students, is not about the power women may hold when their clothing is off, but about how much and what kind power they *retain* once their clothing goes back on.

Taking the risk I'll be misunderstood as prudish, antisexual, or pathetically out of touch, I often share the story about the courthouse with my classes. I want my students to understand that gender in American society is not just personal (as they tend to see it almost exclusively). It's also political. In any culture where men and women and girls and boys are still defined as opposites, and where one gender is constantly depicted as strong, the other, by default, will be relegated to being weak. If our daughters are to be equal and all they deserve to be, they'll need to be smart about gender and power (and sex). One way is to recognize and resist reinforcing stereotypes that ultimately are not in their best interest.

Another sign of blindness among some girls is their superficial ownership of words such as "slut," "bitch," and "'ho." I remember years ago when gay people began to own the word "queer." They took it on proudly, with full awareness and acceptance of its hatefulness, and of the pernicious and rampant hatred of gays throughout society it represented.[6]

Our girls, on the other hand, think words such as "slut" and "bitch," having been neutralized by girls' and women's successes, they assume, are now meaningless. But there is rarely any real step-back and no sense of irony in their using these words so playfully and sometimes proudly to describe themselves or each other, and no real appreciation of how pervasively the sexual double standard is still built into our culture, or how much it can hurt them (even though *at the same time* they complain fiercely to me that boys don't get "reputations" as easily as they). Despite it all, most of them insist there are girls and women who really are "sluts" or "bitches" and who deserve the negative attention they get. They're impervious to the fact that *there is no such thing as "a bitch" or "a slut,"* that these are made-up stereotypes wielded for centuries to keep girls and women in their place. They think all things are now equal because some boys today are called "man whores," without realizing that the referent is still *female*: a "man whore" is a man who's behaving so badly, he's behaving like a woman when she's behaving really, really badly!

Most of all, I want them to get deeply that the only qualification for being called a slut, for real, is being a girl. (Girls don't even have to do anything sexual to invite it; they just have to be a girl.) By keeping the word and the concept alive, girls only ensure that they, their sisters, their cousins, or their best friend could be next. And they also announce to the world, "It's perfectly fine to be unfair to girls. We're okay with that."

Making girls "just as equal" sexually will take hard work—I often leave my middle and high school classes drained and exhausted after these kinds of conversations—but the solution is really pretty simple and straightforward. It's up to adults, especially parents and teachers, to explain that when it comes to sexual values, there's only *one* standard—based on fairness, respect, and caring for and about each other as people—and that it applies absolutely equally both to girls and boys.

Will Boys Be "Boys"?

Three of my seventh-grade students asked me one year if we could view an episode of the Fox TV cartoon show *Family Guy*, called "Emission Impossible," in our human sexuality class. "It's about reproduction," they insisted, "and besides, it's funny." I said I would check it out.

Well, there must be something really wrong with my sense of humor, because most of the episode made me alternately want to scream and cry.

It centers on Stewie, the sexist, foul-mouthed preschooler on the show who hates his mother, fantasizes killing her off in any number of violent ways, and wants to prevent his parents from making a new baby—until he realizes, gleefully, that a new sibling might turn out to be just as nasty as he is. So he sets out to encourage his parents' lovemaking. At one point he peers into their room and tells his dad to "Give it to her good, old man." When his father leaves the bed he orders him to "Come here this instant, you fat bastard, and do her!"

Of course, I know shows like this are intended as farce, but I announced the next day that no, we wouldn't be taking class time to view "Emission Impossible." When I asked my students to guess my reason, they confidently offered suggestions: The language? The women dressed like "bimbos"? The implied sexual acts? The awful treatment of the mother?

"Nope, nope, nope," I replied. "I didn't love any of that, either, but it was the less obvious images and messages that got my attention, the ones that kids your age are clearly less likely to notice. It's not so much that the boy is always acting badly—sometimes that sort of thing can seem so outrageous it's funny. It's the underlying assumption in the show, and often in our society, that boys, by nature, *are bad*."

I said I thought the show's "boys will be bad" message was terribly disrespectful, and I couldn't use our classroom in any way to reinforce it. It was a good moment: recognizing the irony that maybe it was they who were really being demeaned, some of the boys actually got mad.

You can hear and see evidence of this folk "wisdom" about boys almost everywhere, from the gender-typed assumptions people make about young boys to the resigned attitude or blind eye adults so often turn to disrespectful or insensitive male behavior. At the infamous Super Bowl halftime show where Justin Timberlake grabbed at Janet Jackson's breast, it was she who took most of the heat. As the mother of two sons and teacher of thousands of boys, the reaction to that whole incident made me furious, but perhaps not for the reason you may think: I understood it as a twisted kind of compliment to women and a hidden and unfair indictment of men. Was the attitude that it's only women from whom we should expect better behavior?

That incident and so many others explain why, no matter how demeaning today's culture may seem toward girls and women, I've always understood it to be fundamentally *more* disrespectful of boys and men. Consider what "boys will be boys" thinking implies about the true nature of boys. Whenever I ask groups of adults or students what *inherent* traits or characteristics the expression implies, the answers typically are astonishingly negative: boys are messy, immature, and selfish; hormone-driven and insensitive; irresponsible and troublemaking; rebellious, rude, aggressive, and disrespectful—even violent, predatory, and animal-like. Once at a talk I gave, a woman in the audience asked, truly only half in jest, "Is it okay to instruct my daughters that when it comes to sex, teenage boys are animals?"

Adults I work with can easily spot sexism toward girls, yet aren't nearly as savvy about how destructive these same messages can be *for boys*. It often takes patient coaching for them to see "boys will be boys" for what it is, and how insulting it is to imply that poor behavior is what we expect from them.

I think, too, that the staying power of demeaning messages about boys has to do with the fact that as stereotypes go, these can be remarkably invisible.

I've long asked students to bring in print advertisements using sex to sell products or showing people as sex objects. It's no surprise that in the vast majority of ads I receive, women are the focus, not men. But as I try to teach my students, there's always at least one invisible man present in these ads. He's the one supposedly looking at the woman in the image, and he—who's really a stand-in for *every* man—is being stereotyped every bit as much as the women you *can* see. In one example, a magazine ad for a video game, brought to me by a sixth-grade boy, depicts a highly sexualized woman with a dominatrix air brandishing a weapon. The caption reads, "Bet you'd like to get your hands on these!" (meaning her breasts, er, the game controllers). And the man or boy not in the picture, but looking on? Presumably he's just another lowlife guy who lives and breathes to ogle and grab every large-breasted woman he sees.

Many boys I've talked with are pretty savvy about the permission that "boys will be bad" affords and use it to their advantage in their relationships with adults. "Well, they really don't expect as much from us as they do from girls," said one tenth-grade boy. "It makes it easier to get away with a lot of stuff."

Others, sadly, play it sexually to their advantage, knowing that in a system where boys are expected to want sex but not necessarily to be responsible about it, the girl will probably face the consequences if anything happens. As long as girls can still be called sluts, the sexual double standard—and its lack of accountability for boys—will rule.

Most boys I know are grateful when they finally get clued in to all this. A fifth-grade boy once told me that the worst insult anyone could possibly give him would be to call him a girl. When I walked him through what he seemed to be saying—that girls are inferior to him—he was suddenly upset that he could have thought such a thing. "I'm a better person than that," he said.

Just as we've adjusted the bar for girls in academics and athletics, we need to let boys know that in the sexual and social arenas, we've been shortchanging them, too, by setting the bar so low. We need to explain why the notion that "boys will be boys" embodies a bogus set of expectations that are unacceptable. We'll know we've succeeded when girls and boys better recognize sexual and social mistreatment and become angry and personally offended whenever anyone dares use the word "slut" against any girl, call any boy a pimp as a compliment, or suggest that anyone reduce him- or herself or others to a sexual object.

We'll also know when boys call one another more often on disrespectful behavior, instead of being congratulatory, because they will have the self-respect and confidence that comes with being held to and holding yourself to high standards.

In the aftermath of high-profile "boys will be bad" scandals involving high school- and college-age young men, people always say, "We need to teach these boys to have more respect for girls and women." No, I say, we need to show boys more respect, so they'll have more respect for *themselves.*

Most boys do not think, feel, or behave in these ways, though they may go along or remain silent when others do; the social pressures to do so can be enormous. Like my fifth grade students, almost every boy is a good person who deeply understands the importance of kindness, respect, and honesty. The problem is the nearly universal and tacitly accepted cultural attitudes that encourage boys—even give them support and permission—to take a pass on these values when it comes to girls and sex.

All my years of working with kids convinces me how much they appreciate expectations that bring out the very best in who they are. Teenagers as a group are idealistic by nature, a clear indication of their growing intellectual capability to think about matters of right and wrong in terms of abstract, global principles. Teenagers pride themselves on honorable behavior—especially when adults trust and expect them to do the right thing. We may just need to remind them there are no exceptions, especially not when it comes to sex or gender.

Recently a thoughtful high school senior shared with me that he was hopping mad. He had spent some time one afternoon at his girlfriend's house in her room while they studied together (for real). After he left, his girlfriend's mother called her a slut because they had closed the door. What made him even angrier, though, was that she hadn't called him anything. "What?" he said. "She thinks that because I'm a boy, bad behavior is just expected, so what's the use in calling me a name?"

Now there's a young man who deeply gets self-respect. And I have to believe an adult in his life helped him get it.

Reprise: What Does Sexuality Have to Do with Morality?

Here are some examples I use in my high school classes to stretch my students' minds about sexuality and ethics. Most of them—I always toss in some examples of my own—were submitted to me anonymously by students over the years in response to the following prompt: What is a behavior, situation, or decision having to do with sex, gender, or reproduction that you believe is morally wrong? I ask them to work in groups to rank them from "least wrong" to "most wrong" and to decide which ethical values, if any, in their opinion are transgressed in each example.

With younger students, I use more open-ended examples pertinent to their age. I ask them to assign each example to one of three piles ("disapprove," "not sure," "approve") and then ask them to discuss their reasons.

You might try some variation of these activities with your kids at the dinner table. One good way to start is to say you saw these examples in a book you were reading and you're curious about what they think, but then be sure to make up some of your own and/or use some of theirs. Whatever answers they give, simply listen carefully and then ask thought-provoking questions to help them look at things in a different way to stretch their thinking.

Upper Elementary School Examples

- Not sharing your favorite dessert
- Tattling on someone you don't like
- Tattling on a friend
- Saying you left your homework home when you didn't do it at all
- Giving a compliment to get a favor from someone
- Hiding someone's book bag for fun
- Telling a fib to keep a friend out of trouble
- Telling an adult that your friend secretly makes herself throw up in the bathroom
- Inviting everyone in your class to a party except for two people you don't like
- Sitting with popular kids instead of your friend at lunch
- Having a "boyfriend" or "girlfriend" in the fifth grade
- Going on a "date" in the fifth grade

Middle School Examples

- Breaking up with someone in an e-mail
- Kissing somebody at a party
- Looking at pornography
- Teasing a boy often by saying he's really a girl
- Spreading rumors about someone who is really mean to people
- Staying up late to text your friends
- Talking with your friends about particular girls' or boys' bodies
- Watching a movie at a friend's house that your parents would not want you to see
- Forwarding an e-mail that puts down another student at school
- Using lots of raunchy language when adults aren't around
- Saying yes to a kiss because you want the other person to like you
- Trying to take away another person's boyfriend or girlfriend you really like

High School Examples

- Two eleventh-grade boys hitting on a ninth grader
- Two eleventh-grade girls hitting on a ninth grader
- Aborting a fetus for gender selection
- Putting a hand back on a breast or genital after the other person has moved it away
- Having intercourse with someone you just met
- Having a vasectomy behind your wife's back
- Not using protection against an unwanted pregnancy and/or sexually transmitted infections
- Making out with your friend's boyfriend or girlfriend
- Repeatedly calling someone at school a "fag," "slut," or "'ho" (purposeful insult, not a "joke")
- Saying "that's so gay" whenever and wherever you feel like it
- Prostitution (I like to leave this one open-ended)
- Sending nude cell phone pictures of an ex-girlfriend
- Lying to someone (e.g., saying "I really like you") to get a sexual favor

"Okay/Not Okay/Not Sure"

Question to ask: What is your opinion about the following reasons for saying "yes" to a kiss?

- For fun
- To be physically close
- To see what it's like
- To show affection or love
- To feel more grown up
- For pleasure
- To get the person to like you
- To be able to say "I did it"

Follow Up: What reasons are okay or not okay for other sexual experiences? Which ones are "good enough" reasons and which ones aren't "good enough" on their own? Why or why not?

7

The Delicate Art
of Limit Setting

ere's a scary story for you. A few years ago, a middle school principal called me for some help. The place was in recovery mode over an incident earlier in the week, when two eighth graders were discovered engaging in oral sex—on an open stairway, no less. It was *after* school, they explained, so wasn't that okay?

And that's not the scary part!

Rumors were flying, and the school made the decision to talk with students about the incident in its characteristically up-front way. Administrators notified parents, and teachers received training in how to conduct discussion with their mixed advisory groups of sixth, seventh, and eighth graders. The conversations went exceptionally well, because the school works hard to provide a safe, nurturing environment, and kids trust adults to provide helpful guidance around real-life issues of all kinds. Teachers are unafraid to take any bull by the horns, no matter how sharp (or sexual), if it will help their students thrive.

As the kids filed out of the group that I led, a sixth-grade boy stopped to say, "Thanks for coming. I just thought you *had* to have sex in middle school. I wouldn't have known different if we didn't have this talk."

He looked decidedly relieved, as you can imagine. "I'm curious: How come you thought that?" I asked. "Well," he said, "there was a big story on the cover of the newspaper a couple of weeks ago. It said, 'Oral Sex in Middle School.'"[1]

We forget, don't we, just how literally children take in the world as it rolls on by. And this was a plain old black-and-white newspaper sitting out on the kitchen table! Imagine what conclusions kids are, at every turn, drawing from the glitzy, sensationalized media looking to pull in their eyes. This boy was almost twelve. *What about all those third graders,* I thought, *their antennae stretched high, searching for clues about what makes adult society tick.* I recalled something my eight-year-old son said once about his best friend's two-month-old baby brother. When I mentioned his mother was nursing him, my son adamantly said: "Oh, no, that baby isn't nursing *yet.* Have you seen his mouth? It isn't big enough yet!" (If they'd named it "nipple feeding" instead of "breast feeding" my son would've understood just fine.)

An Internet-savvy seventh grader once sent me a link to a "real" credit card advertisement he'd found online. A boy and girl are standing at the front door of her house kissing after a date. He says to her, "How about a 'blow job'?" to which she replies, "Are you crazy? My parents are inside." The volley continues until the girl's sister finally comes down and opens the door. "Dad says to give him the 'blow job' already so we can all get some sleep," she relays, and then instructs the boy to move his elbow off the intercom button. The punch line at the end: "Your girlfriend's father having a really good sense of humor: priceless."

Since then, I always describe this "commercial" to my seventh-grade classes and ask them to vote (anonymously) on whether they think it's a real ad or not, and then to justify their choice in discussion. In the end, the groups are usually split half and half, "real" and "not real," with most kids saying, actually, they could go either way. Their lack of "step-back" is blatant; they simply don't have the life experience or mental processing skills to ask themselves the right questions about what they see. It reminds me of the time a sixth grader vehemently insisted in class that a woman should use whatever she can, including her sex appeal, to get ahead on the job. When I wondered how she thought that worked in the real world, where women need and want their work to be taken seriously, she asked if I meant the *Real World* on MTV or the other one.

By the way, about half my seventh graders, too, take me seriously when I tell them that I'll be standing behind a screen at their high school graduation, and unless they can recite, word for word, the five-part definition of a hormone I've just taught them, they can't get their diploma on stage. The other half are pretty sure I'm kidding, but they look like they're not going to take any chances. Don't think for a second that marketers don't know how gullible they are, too.

Given their cognitive shortcomings, normal as they are, children and early adolescents belong in a world tailored for them, and not a boundary-free universe of limitless possibilities they can't possibly process correctly or well. But to paraphrase a former US secretary of defense, in a very different context, you raise your kids in the world you have, not in the world you wish you had. It's us our children look to first, regardless of what *that* world looks like. Always keep that in mind.

Wearing "the Suit"

Just before the turn of the new century, I started hearing rumbles of a new trend that school people I know across the country were starting to see. "What is it with parents today?" they kept asking. "They're just not getting this limit-setting thing."

More than a decade later, I hear that from large numbers of parents, too. Many describe feeling as if they're the only ones who put their foot down or say no to their kids—about electronics, media, Internet access, e-mail, cell phones, texting, social networking, curfews, privileges, expensive and revealing clothing, dating, you name it. They're beleaguered, and they're angry, frustrated that other parents make it so hard for them to do their job. One dad said to me recently, "There are three kinds of parents: the ones who get it, the ones who don't, and the ones who get it but are too afraid of their own kids to do anything about it."

Regardless of trends, and this one definitely rings true, I always encourage parents—and school people—to be cautious about generalizing. Sometimes parents describe themselves as the "choir" I'm preaching to, and say it's the parents who don't come who need to. I like to tease them back: "Hey, you're here, and they're home parenting. Guess what they say about you!" I will, though, always commit myself to the principle that clear limits and boundaries aren't just *nice* or *good* for children and teens; they're bedrock. Without them youngsters are lost, and left to fend for themselves in a world too big for them to step back and see whole, let alone safely manage. Though meeting all five of children's needs is vital, doing well with the other four may be for naught if we don't see to their safety first.

So, What Is It with Parents Today?

To the degree parents act as if limits don't matter, there will likely be costs. Some years ago, I read about a group of eighth graders who, it was discovered, were meeting in various locations—indoor and out—to engage in oral sex with one another. The story caused near panic, fed by media coverage about an "epidemic" among young teens. (Teenage sex sells—beware what you read.) I had only one question at the time: Where were the parents? Whenever kids are coloring that far out of the lines, adults are way too out of touch.

Simply put, limits aren't "optional" for our kids, they're *oxygen.* So, indeed, "What is it with some parents today?"

I am certain the factors are numerous, and many in fact have healthy roots. For one, since the 1960s, people in general live lives increasingly casual in tone, and when young people become adults they don't see themselves as "authority figures" on high nearly as before. People of all ages mix and mingle in all kinds of ways today. There is a family I and my husband are close to, and when we're all together I can't figure out what generation I'm in, much less anyone else. The man is eight years my senior, but his wife, a former student of mine, is ten years younger than I; his children from a previous marriage are years older than our children, but he and his present wife have kids twenty years younger than ours, and their children and his grandchildren are pretty close in age. Amazingly, none of it seems to matter. When any combination of us is together, we just consider ourselves dear friends who care about one another a lot.

Informality can breed lots of good feelings and togetherness, but there's a downside for kids whose parents don't fully grasp that they are parents first, last, and always. We can be very friendly toward our kids and enjoy those moments to the fullest, but that's not at all the same thing as being "friends." Like Superman in a phone booth (what's a phone booth?), parents must be ready, at a second's notice, to switch into their parenting and boundaries "suit" and take on their roles. That's very hard to do when the ground rules are mush. It's clear, too, that marketers know just how to further blur the boundaries between kids and adults—on both sides of the equation: Marketing youth to adults and adulthood to youths is big business. And as I wrote in Chapter 2, this is the first generation of parents to contend with multibillion-dollar corporations wheedling their way in between them and their kids.

Drama is part of every preteen's and teenager's repertoire. Most often when they say things like, "I hate you! My social life will be *over* if you won't let me go," they genuinely believe in the moment that it's true. Their anguish is so real and so convincing, parents may come to think so, too. These are some of the hardest situations in which to keep our cool and our resolve, and to stay separate enough that we don't "catch" their overblown feelings and lose our perspective. We have to be willing for our children to "hate" us sometimes; it probably means we're doing our job. And besides, if we remember who has the real power in the family and who owns all the "stuff," it won't take them long to realize they need us too much to hate us for long.

If parenting indeed were a "five-piece suit," limit-setting would definitely be the pants (especially now that both women and men wear them). A well-pressed pair of pants with a decided crease communicates, "I'm to be taken seriously, no matter what else I might wear."

Artful Limit-Setting

Way back in Chapter 3, I described limits as brackets we put around our children to keep them safe and healthy. I especially appreciate the way Lori Radun a life coach and parent educator, expands that idea.[2] Lori views boundaries as our sacred protectors in life, and limits as actions we take to keep our boundaries intact, so we don't get "used up" or give ourselves away. She contends that a healthy and successful life requires us to actively protect our boundaries around seven things: our bodies, self-worth, time, space, money, energy, and relationships. (There's lots related to sexuality in that list, isn't there?) Setting limits for children goes way beyond saying no, she says. It's about helping kids learn how to protect and best use their precious resources—and how to respect others'—in the service of a good life. Interesting, huh?

And for sure, sometimes what's called for is a simple and resounding no. We can't forget, though, that as parents we teach and communicate way more about limits and their importance by what we do and what we model than by what we say. Our tone of voice and its firmness (or not), our consistency, our actions (from baby-proofing the living room to physically removing a screaming child to physically removing the car keys or the Internet access), and our facial expressions—you should see the deadly "seventh-grade stare" I've perfected—tell our kids much more than mere words. So do narrowing our kids' choices to a realistic, safe, and manageable number, and perhaps most important of all, unflinching follow-through to prove that, yes, limits do exist. We can lay out our expectations for kids beautifully, and think of great and logical consequences if they're not met, but unless we impose them fearlessly, kids won't take us or them seriously. Like I tell my students, you haven't really done your homework unless you actually bring it with you to school.

But *Where* to Put Them?

As always, the key to responsive parenting is knowing who your children are, as unique individuals *and* from the perspective of developmental stage. *How children think* at different ages and stages is the least visible but often the most reliable guide for setting safe and reasonable limits around their behavior and choices. If you're sensing the need to keep a fairly tight rein on a child's freedom, her or his cognitive ability—not only her or his level of social or emotional maturity—is a good reason.

We accept that younger children need a watchful adult eye, but things can get hairy when they're too big for babysitters, yet too young to manage real independence on their own. An eleven- or twelve-year-old's thought process, for example, can seem deceptively mature. As concrete thinkers, risk-taking to them is a black-and-white affair: if something bad *could* happen, in their mind it *will*. You shouldn't use drugs, they'll tell you, because drugs *will* kill you. Don't have sexual intercourse, because you *will* get a sexually transmitted infection (and die), because you *will* get pregnant. You won't die from pregnancy, but when your parents find out, they'll kill you. Somehow the story always ends up with death.

Though they may seem convincingly cautious, these are not young people to be trusted with weighty decisions. Since they don't yet think in the abstract realm of "might," they often grossly overestimate—or just as easily, grossly underestimate—the risks inherent in their choices. Soon enough, though, at about age thirteen, a capacity for thinking more realistically about future events begins to emerge: "If I do *x*, there's a good chance I'll get into trouble, but if I do *y* or *z*, I can get what I want without running that risk." But their reasoning still will take them only so far. I once heard someone aptly refer to kids' thinking at this stage as adolescent *almost* logic: if a thirteen- or fourteen-year-old has at least one good reason for doing or not doing something, especially if she believes it's a really, *really* good one, it's often enough. It simply may not occur to her to think any further; all the "yes, buts" a more sophisticated mind might stop to entertain won't even seem relevant. Even if they did, other more immediate social or emotional risks in the moment—not some invisible and hypothetical consequence off in the future—might easily prevail. That's why kids this age need freedom and space to grow, but always with a brightly painted fence around it.

Once they are in high school, teenagers' ability to look into the immediate and longer-term future, and to consider possibilities, probabilities, and likely outcomes of their choices, strengthens each year. But so do the demands and challenges they face. Ever-changing social expectations, and the parade of brand-new situations they continuously confront, test these new capacities to the max. Throw alcohol or other drugs into the mix, and what they know and how skillfully they can think may not matter. As I'm always telling my students, the first effect alcohol has on the brain, even in lower doses, is to inhibit the part that causes you to second-guess your decisions. (That's the flip side of why it's such an effective "social lubricant"; under the influence, we don't second-guess what we're about to say nearly as much.) It's no mystery why alcohol or other drugs is the number-one co-factor present in cases of unprotected sexual intercourse and date or acquaintance rape.

There's another feature of normal adolescence that makes it tough to know how much supervision our teenagers need. In an ironic developmental twist, teens' intellect and their beliefs don't always match up. They know certain behaviors are risky but may believe *they personally* are immune: "The laws of probability apply to everyone else, but not me." According to psychologist David Elkind, many teens spin this "personal fable" about their own invincibility as a defense against the anxiety, even terror, associated with separating from parents and taking control of their own lives. It's something they grow out of, but at their own individualized pace; a select group of teens socializing together could be all over this developmental map. The "stupid" decisions they may make, or go along with, may not be about intellect at all. And for some, not even a really close call, or an awful consequence resulting from a poor decision, will shake them out of their denial if they're not developmentally ready. Like getting a first period, it happens when it happens and not a day before. Keep in mind, too, that some kids at this stage believe, conversely, that potential risks *overly* apply to them: "If something bad will happen, it's going to happen to *me.*" Those kids may suffer from the effects of refusing to take risks that might well be an important asset to their development, and they need our encouragement.

With the advancement of brain science in recent years has come a spate of fascinating studies on the teen brain. There's now ample evidence to suggest that teens' emotional volatility, impulsivity, and propensity to engage in, and even to seek out, risky behaviors are associated with *normal changes* in how the brain functions and matures during these years.[3] With their psychology and biology working at cross purposes to rational decision-making, even as their intellectual development advances, teens need adults who continue to be vigilant about supervision and monitoring.

Cognitive Development Is One of Your Best Guides

There's no way around it, and there's no parental reprieve: babies need cribs; older kids need freedom with a fence around it; and high school kids need guardrails, at least (so do college kids). They all need adults who remember that no matter how smart or how tall, how responsible or how relatively mature for their age, they don't think like us. It's wise to keep tabs on how they do think and reason, at every age and stage, for the best clues about which kind of boundaries—cribs, fences, or guardrails—they need.[4]

Here, for example, are three simple tests. (1) Ask your twelve-year-old, "What does the expression 'The grass is always greener on the other side of the fence' mean?" If he or she says, "It means they have a lawn service," you've still got a concrete thinker on your hands. (2) If your eighth grader can't think up three potential consequences of a particular decision, and two consequences of each of those consequences, and how likely each is to happen, make sure he or she is supervised closely. (3) If your eleventh grader wants to go on an out-of-town excursion and says, "Don't worry. Everything will be fine," don't buy it without a conversation. Insist she come up with at least three unexpected things that could happen, and contingencies for each. If she can't, or won't, keep the keys (then refer her to the section below, "Independence Is Earned").

The Adolescent Law of Limit-Setting

Everybody knows about the law of gravity, and that it works every single time. I'm a thirty-plus-year teacher, with tens of thousands of classroom hours, and I know this law to be almost as dependable. Really!

All adolescents need and want limits, and they are at their very best when adults place the boundaries "just so." I know this for sure because of what I see in my classrooms every day. If I'm unclear about my role or expectations, my students are likely to test and test, sometimes until I actually have to yell, *"Stop!"* On the other hand, if I don't cut them *enough* slack and they feel too constrained, they'll typically push back then, too. But on days when I hit just the right balance of clear structure and wide-open range, the class is literally transformed; we enter a bubble or "zone"—not unlike what runners describe— where learning takes off at an exhilarating pace. It's a joy to behold, and the best kind of fun a teacher can have. It's why teachers love teaching.

Americans tend to stereotype teenagers as naturally rebellious. Not necessarily so! They typically rebel only when there's something concrete to rebel against. If rules are plainly unfair or hypocritical, or fail to realistically take into account teens' changing needs and capacities, they may decide the rules aren't worth following, and neither is the person (or institution) who tried to imposed them. They also may push, and push hard, if our limits are way off base—in either direction.

If parents are way too laissez-faire, some kids actually will do something pretty outrageous, if not out-and-out dangerous, that's guaranteed to gain their attention (attention = love), hoping at least unconsciously to get their parents to parent. Others, hemmed in too long by limits that don't reflect their need to grow, may begin flagrantly to violate family rules, or lie about their activities, or sneak around behind their parents' backs. In extreme cases, they may even take part of themselves away to an underground life parents know nothing about. Remember, too, that inexperienced teens may simply not know the point beyond which certain behaviors become danger- ous, sort of like those poor, clueless goldfish that don't know when to stop eating and eventually overfeed themselves to death.

Striking a balance, and tweaking it as necessary, makes limit-setting the art that it is; think of it as calibrating a radio station that's fuzzy to start and fades in and out as you drive down the highway. Expect trial and error, and if you're really unsure, check in with a counselor or another parent you know who has been there and done that well.

Here's a predictable truth: if you get it just right or as close as you're able, kids still may test your rules—to show you (and them) they can—but for the most part they won't test too far. Kids who've been taught explicitly to un- derstand why limits and boundaries are important in life don't resent their parents for setting them nearly as much as kids who haven't. And by the way, since the adolescent law of limit-setting almost always works, if there are sit- uations where you absolutely don't want your children to test your rules be- yond a certain point, you can always set the limit *just inside* where you think it belongs. (You might want to tear out this page and eat it now before your kids catch on.)

Adolescents need to know that we still think of limits as part of our job and that our expectations are simply part of the family landscape, not some dia- bolical plan to frustrate them or keep them from having fun. It's only fair, and smart, to let them know up front that we will make misjudgments—usually on the side of caution—but that we're adaptable and truly happy to grant more freedom once we're convinced it's okay. And we need to constantly do our homework: Where are they going? What will they do? Is it within their developmental range? Who will be watching out for them and their friends, and how?

It's unfortunate, and ironic, that once teenagers and their peers start to drive, parents tend to pull back, just when kids' independence takes off exponentially (and when, statistically, alcohol and other drug use among teenagers dramatically increases). Mistake! When older teens get the idea their parents no longer care as much about limits, or seem to have just thrown in the towel, they're likely to conclude it means they're mature enough to handle *anything*—and I do mean that literally—that might come their way. Not yet so. When we're on top of risks and limits—around parties, alcohol and other drug use, sexual behavior, drinking and driving or riding, etc.—there's a much better chance they will make safer and more considered choices. Decades of research back up that fact.

Staying actively involved reminds them, at least, that there *are* limits to freedom in all parts of life, even when they're just trying to have a good time. After a talk at a parochial high school in New York, I was chatting with some parents about their kids when two juniors, there to write an article for the school newspaper, approached us. "What you said was okay," the girl came to tell me, "but none of it matters. Teenagers are going to do what they want to do, and there's nothing parents can or should do to stop them. They'll just have to trust us to make our own decisions and mistakes."

The boy with her nodded approvingly, glad she was setting us straight. The parents were done in by all this, you could tell, but kept their cool. They were worried, they said, because teenagers aren't yet adults and don't always have the wisdom to make the best choices, and that some of those choices could be dangerous. "That doesn't matter," the boy said, miffed they couldn't see the absolute truth in what he and the girl were saying. "At our age we're entitled to do stupid things, even if they're harmful." "Entitled to increasing freedom, definitely," said one dad. "But no one is *entitled* to hurt himself or other people." The fine distinction was lost on them both, another good reason not to back off just yet.

Teenagers, itching for independence and feeling constrained by what they can't yet do, typically define freedom, understandably, as doing what you want, whenever you want to do it. That's one kind of freedom—freedom from restraint—but it's not nearly the whole story. If you only do what you want to do, I'm always reminding them, ultimately you'll end up with *fewer* degrees of freedom in the future. Real freedom isn't *freedom from* anything; it's the *freedom to* make responsible choices that support your well-being (and the well-being of others) and *increase* your options and freedom going forward. Freedom without responsibility isn't really freedom at all. It's license.

Independence Is Earned

"The media" is everywhere, and we simply take it for granted most of the time. In reality of course it's not the monolith that nickname implies. There are all kinds of media and all kinds of content, much of it of course containing sexual messages, both embedded and overt. Calvin Klein ads frankly don't bother me nearly as much as others that are blatantly sexist or dehumanizing even though everyone's clothes are *on*. Those are the ones, actually, I suggest we pay attention to most with our kids: "Do you see how that woman is kneeling at the man's feet, waiting, it seems, for his next command? He looks like a king sitting there, and that lacrosse stick in his hand looks like a scepter he might actually hit her with if she doesn't obey. Wait, isn't that the company's logo tattooed on her back?"

As for movies, games, and TV programming, as I've said earlier, whatever we can control, we should, for as long as we can. For kids whose natural "stepback" capacity is next to nil (for most, that's clear through fifth grade), I'm all for banishing anything we're not certain is truly geared toward children. And I know just how hard that can be—surely Ted Geisel, the beloved Dr. Seuss, is still rolling over in his grave about the adult sexual references in the movie *The Cat in the Hat*—but vigilance is well worth the effort. It's essential for this age group, to protect them and also to give us time to get there first.

When my son was five years old, a dog stepped on his toe. He looked at the dog sternly and said, "That was not appropriate." It was then I realized I just might be overusing that word. Especially when setting limits around what we consider too grown-up for young kids to watch or listen to because of its sexual content, it's a really good idea to say something other than "You can't see that because it's not appropriate." Without further explanation, many kids surmise we're saying *sex itself* is inappropriate, or even that it's bad. What we need, and I think, mean, to communicate is about *context*, not sex: "That movie has things in it about sex. It's really important to learn about that subject in the right way, and it's our job to teach you. That movie will give you wrong or confusing ideas about sex that we don't want you to have."

When it comes to young adolescents, there's virtually no chance they won't be exposed to popular media—through other kids' chatter, Internet sites, magazines, news sources, and/or exposure to media at another child's home. No matter how hard we might try to curtail their exposure, the law of diminishing returns eventually takes hold. But don't throw up your hands in despair, or feel out of control. You need only shift gears. This is exactly the right time to step up your efforts to cultivate your children's media literacy skills. Once they start paying attention to a wider world, it means—within limits—they also have a sharper ability, with help, to process what they see.

This is also one of those moments when wearing the pants in the family really pays off. "Child," you can say, "you know those two movies you've been wanting to see that Dad and I decided were too advanced for you? Well, today is your lucky day, and I'll give you your ticket: we're going to watch them together, and here are the rules." (You'll of course want to preview the movies first on your own to make sure they're not too far over the top, and so you can get your thoughts together.) After viewing the first one, turn to your son or daughter and identify each and every scene that concerned you and precisely why. After the second film, turn to him or her and say, "Now *you* tell *me* all the things I didn't like about that one." Repeat the process as often as you think necessary, until you're convinced that, indeed, your children have your lens over their eyes and your voice in their head. (They don't have to agree with you, remember, just know how to think like you.) Each time they pass your test, they get more freedom in choosing what they want to view. You'll be amazed and proud that soon enough they'll see things that escaped your eyes entirely.

What's more, you'll have reinforced a principle that will serve you and them well in all kinds of situations: "In this family, independence—the ability to choose what you do on your own—isn't an entitlement, it's earned."

By the way, suppose they can't pass your test. Well, that's part of the process, too. Just tell them you are *always* available for a retest.

Your kids will eventually get to an age—probably sixteen at the latest—when control over much of their media exposure will become practically (in both senses of the word) impossible. But here's the hope: by that time, they won't need any more tests.

Holding On to Your Power and
Authority (or At Least Not Giving It Away)

Every parent needs and deserves a mentor. Once your child reaches double digits, or before if it will help, find yourself a person who will take you on as a kind of, let's say, community service project. Promise to take him or her out for coffee, lunch, or dinner (or all three!) once a month and help you stay ahead of your kids and the dizzying pace of development to come. Choose someone who's a strong, fair, and responsive limit-setter, and whose non-perfect children (who sometimes cross well-drawn lines) like and respect their parents a lot nonetheless.

Whenever news breaks about some teenage sex "revelation" (think: hooking up, friends with benefits, sexting, threesomes, orgies), many parents become totally flummoxed. I remember especially when the first newspaper stories appeared about oral sex and young teens in the early 2000s. I received calls from reporters who were oddly speechless; in a very weird twist, I found myself having to frame the questions, not simply answer them. I saw seasoned radio interviewers throw up their hands during commercial breaks and exclaim, "I can't believe this!" They just couldn't find their objectivity, I suppose because they kept thinking about their own kids or grandkids.

We don't ever want to be that out of touch even with the possibilities that exist in our children's world. That's what a savvy mentor can do for you: keep you abreast of what might come up in the weeks and months ahead so you'll hardly ever be blindsided by what you hear from or about your kids and their friends.

If you have children up through age nine, here's a splendid way to celebrate their birthdays each year. Find a good resource to help you brush up on the unique characteristics—physical, social, emotional, and intellectual—of children that age. That way you'll know going in what to expect of them as children, and of you as the parent of a child in this stage. (It will also convince you, on challenging days, that, yup, they're just normal, and this too shall pass.) Once they turn ten, though, you'll need to begin educating yourself about development that year *and the next year.* Until then, changes in parenting are generally smooth and incremental, but parenting an eleven-year-old, and so on, is going to be cosmically different from year to year. Becoming an expert on your child's development six months to a year ahead of time is a great way to stay out in front of your child's social and emotional world. It also maximizes the opportunities to build in capacities your child will need this year *and* next, and to give *yourself* plenty of anticipatory guidance about the kind of parent you'll need to be then.

Here's an example of how unprepared parents may unwittingly give away chunks of their power: Your daughter is *begging* you to go to a party. You don't know the parents, or most of the kids who will be there. She names two kids you know who are going, but you're unimpressed and say so. Then she says, "But, Dad, Devon is going!" You say to yourself, *Devon? Devon is going? Devon's mom is a terrific parent. It must be okay.* The minute you say yes, it is now Devon's mom, not you, who is parenting your child. (It doesn't even matter, by the way, whether Devon's mom is your mentor.) Our kids need to know we will do our own independent research before we make up our minds, even if it's one quick call.

And another example: Suppose it's October and your son has recently entered middle school. It's a Friday night, you're in the kitchen, and he and some old friends, who've been congregating in your basement for years, plus a few kids he has just met at his new school, are downstairs. Something feels different, though, than last year; either the music's so loud you can't hear anything else, or it's eerily quiet, except for loud outbursts of laughter. You're a little concerned. You think about going downstairs but don't want to embarrass your son in front of his new friends. Then you realize you don't really know anything about these new kids, and moreover, when his old friends bounced in the door, some looked decidedly older. You now start wringing your hands. But after a few minutes of pacing and imagining the worst, you say to yourself, *Nah—they're the same adorable, levelheaded kids I've known, well, forever. Everything is probably fine. Stop worrying.*

The minute you decide—despite your instincts—not to go check things out, you've sent your young son the message that *he's* the one in charge of his social life, and of you and your home. Whenever kids are socializing in your house, it's simply your *adult presence*—defined as kids' knowing you could show your face literally at any moment—that will keep them in check. What even a brief appearance communicates is, "There are limits in this house."

As hard as it may be to stick to your guns, if your children insist you can't just drop by, well, it's time to affirm their disappointment and then say, "Sorry, no party." Besides, you can always come up with creative ways to "show your face" that won't be intrusive but will do the trick. For example, when kids are coming over, here's what I suggest: Lock up the liquor, any weapons you may own, and all cabinets that contain large-size bowls. Then go out to the store, buy inexpensive *small* bowls, and bags of very salty food. Keep the beverages and food refills in the kitchen, or in whichever room you just happen to be. Or if you've moved your washer and dryer upstairs, and kids socialize downstairs, move them back down! That way you can save up your laundry, and dash in and out. All kidding aside (you know I don't really mean you have to move the washer, right?), of course the best creative solutions are the ones you and your child cook up together. Once a bargain is struck, you'll get to supervise, and she'll get to have you as invisible as possible.

In giving your children a voice in what goes, learn to think and act like a negotiator, and prime yourself for compromise. If your eighth grader, for example, wants to invite twenty kids to a party, you might lowball your opening bid somewhere around ten. Fifteen will come to feel like a victory for you both. Or, as your ninth grader begins to value her independence ever more acutely, honest and respectful give-and-take will honor her growing capacity to make sound decisions and also will keep you in the loop. Overtly establishing your expectations at the outset works very effectively, too. Children: as you mature, you will have increasing say in the limits we set, *and* (not "but") we're going to remain the ultimate "deciders" about certain things while you are still under our roof, such as putting schoolwork, health, family time, religious observance, or other important things first. Make it explicit, too, that issues of safety will always be nonnegotiable and that you won't hesitate to pull back on their freedom when you think they're at risk. Bottom line: when teenagers, clear through high school, know the rules and expectations ahead of time and are helped to see their importance, at least from your point of view, they are typically much less resistant to your rules.

At some point almost all teens break an important rule or otherwise violate your trust. Those situations, even if they precipitate a crisis of sorts in the family, most often lead to important learning and growth. A particularly worrisome situation can arise when teens feel they're in danger or want a way out, but they've lied to you about where they are or about the activities they're involved in. My advice to *all* families is to agree to a "no questions asked until tomorrow" rule. Kids need to know they can summon you with a preplanned signal at any time, no matter the location or circumstance, and you will pick them up immediately without comment. The conversation will happen, and logical consequences may be imposed, but not until tomorrow.

A word to the wise, in the "picking your battles" department: try not to put your foot down too hard over behaviors you probably can't control, or in a situation where you might not have the resolve to carry through. Otherwise you stand to compromise your credibility on other matters, too. It's not good policy to label a behavior "intolerable" when, if you're honest with yourself, you know you'll probably continue to tolerate it. So, before you're about to create a battle royal with one of your kids, decide whether it's one you can actually win. Unless the issue is safety, in which case you're the one in charge, a strong statement of disapproval, said firmly once or twice, may be your best approach. Speaking of disapproval, there's a body of research that demonstrates it's effective. Kids are less likely to engage in risky behaviors beyond parents' direct control when parents express their disapproval, and give specific and sensible reasons.

It Is Easier to Ride a Horse in the Direction in Which It's Going

Many parents complain that their eighth, ninth, or tenth grader suddenly starts talking in monosyllables. Getting any information out of them at all about their day, their social life, their goals, their interests, you name it, seems next to impossible. Though sudden changes in behavior among adolescents are sometimes red flags—a precipitous drop in grades, abrupt switches in friendship groups, withdrawal from friends or favorite activities—this one is typical of normal "pulling in and away." Even so, the new sounds of silence make a lot of parents understandably nervous; cut off from almost all reassuring tidbits, they easily imagine the worst. And of course, the more they press for information, the more their kids typically withhold.

If you remember to wear your "suit," and stay in touch with your power, this situation can be an opportunity, not a dead end. First, scale down your expectations to a "need to know" basis, and let the rest ride for at least a while. The mental "scale-down" process is a good exercise in itself. Then pick a time in your family when everyone is happy with everyone. (Don't laugh.) Knock on your son's or daughter's door and ask to come in because you have some really good advice. Calmly, and in a matter-of-fact way, say something like:

> You know, it's very clear that you want a lot more independence than before. I'm not unhappy with that at all—you need to grow up and away from us. And [not "but"] at the same time, I'm still responsible for you and your safety. So let me tell you up front how things are going to work. The more information you give us (right now I need to know more about x, y, and z), the more quickly I'll be willing to grant the increasing independence you want so badly, and we really want to give you. Of course the opposite is also true. The less information I have now and going forward, the slower the process will happen. The choice is entirely up to you. Dinner's in ten.

That last sentence, followed immediately by your exiting the room, is the most important part. This is not going to be a *conversation,* because what you've said is simply not negotiable, and you don't have to defend it. Since the desire for independence is the direction teenagers are already going in, if we're smart about development we can use this (and other) normal characteristic of mid-adolescence to their advantage *and* ours by not resisting it but guiding it. You and they need to know that you're not the police, you're a nurturer.

Parenting Is Definitely Not a One-Family Job

So often today I meet parents who tell me, "I'm at my wits' end. I've tried everything with my kids, all the things the 'experts' say to do, but the demands they make and the stuff they're exposed to and want me to buy gets the best of me. What else can I do?"

Honestly, as I hate to tell them, there's probably little else they can do. Their frustration, I say, comes from trying to solve a problem they simply cannot solve on their own, because parenting today is not a one-family job.[5] There's no magic bullet they've missed or ever will find. Parents help themselves best by recognizing they cannot do this job alone, no matter how many books they read or lectures they go to or how hard they try. The most effective buffer against the tsunami of popular culture is still "the village." Parents need and deserve—and so do their children—the support of other parents within their communities. *What will make an appreciable difference in their lives is creating an alliance with like-minded parents who can provide one another ongoing reinforcement, support, and ideas.*

Whether through informal networking or organized grade-level meetings at school, parents can help one another by taking stock and comparing notes, particularly about safe and age-appropriate limit-setting. They can also take a page out of their children's own playbook. Parents, too, can use texting, video conferencing, and social networking for check-ins. Though it won't work well if kids feel hounded or under surveillance—I'd be really low-key about checking in with other parents, and try hard not to throw it in kids' faces in any way—just the fact that parents are in communication lets them know adults are paying attention. Besides, when your kids insist you're the *only* parent east of the Mississippi (or west, depending on where you live) who won't let them do or buy something they want, you can smile (inwardly) and mention the names of parents you know who've agreed to say no, too. Eventually your kids will "get it"—that you and other parents are all wearing the "suit," all the time—and their whining will diminish because they'll know there's no point.

Stellar research demonstrates that kids' beliefs[6] about who among their peers is doing, or is buying, or is allowed to do what are usually grossly inflated. Kids have far-off-the-mark beliefs about older kids' behaviors, too, so that when they think about next year or the year after, or even beyond, they anticipate (incorrectly) what "everyone is doing" and what they'll have to do, too. The entertainment media encourage these false perceptions by putting scene after scene in front of kids' faces where all or almost all the teen characters are taking potentially dangerous risks.

Researchers conclude that kids' distorted "normative beliefs" about risky behaviors among teens significantly drive the actual incidence of unhealthy behaviors *upward*. In reality, it's the kids in any community who make healthy decisions who are in the decided majority, not the ones who don't. Starting in elementary school, when parents work together to educate one another about what's really going on, and not, in their children's peer group (starting with bedtimes, allowance, clothing, purchases, cell phones, Internet use, electronics, TV, movies, socializing, etc.), they can keep their kids' normative beliefs in a realistic ballpark. Clear through high school, they can become a united force against corporate interests and behaviors that can harm.

Parents also have to be willing to face the peer pressure they want their children to resist. Calling other parents to check things out can be really hard, especially if you start out with something like, "Hello. My son is coming over to play. Are there any guns in the home?" The trick is to always talk about yourself first: "I'm calling to say I'm glad our children are friends and I hope he'll come over often. I want you to know the rules in our home, and the kinds of supervision we provide, so you'll always feel good about your child coming to our house. And because we like to be consistent about limits, I'm hoping you'll share the rules at your house, too." If you're not comfortable with what you hear, play dates or socializing can happen at your house, not theirs.

Imagine the power they would hold if all parents could and would make these kinds of calls. For those in the minority who don't supervise closely enough, or perhaps at all, the word would be out that they are just that, the minority. And best of all, kids wouldn't ever be able to say, "You're the only father east of the Mississippi . . ."

Technology: Taming the Beast

When the latest iPad came out, I got a spate of calls from upset parents, whose stories were very much the same. All had brought their new gadget home and at some point nonchalantly handed it off to a super-excited elementary school–age child. Within a day or two, all four of the children either stumbled onto a website with pornographic images or, in two cases, deliberately sought one out. One eight-year-old boy, it turned out, went to a site "recommended" by another boy his age at school. Practically each parent said the same thing to me: "What was I thinking?" One immediately answered her own question: "I wasn't; that was the problem."

Don't Think of an Elephant[7] is the name of a book written by the linguist George Lakoff. The point of the title is that everyone has "semantic" frames built into his or her mind, created by repeated exposure to specific people, places, things, and ideas in the world. For example, when we see a huge gray mammal with great big ears and a trunk on its face, our brain instantly recognizes the image as "elephant." Picture one now. Now picture another one, but don't think of an elephant as you do. Next to impossible, right?

Computers, cell phones, tablets, and other technological devices have become our constant and sometimes favored companions. They are like magical friends, delivering connectedness, knowledge, entertainment, fun, work, convenience, commerce, visuals, sounds, cameras, and an infinite and instantaneous array of other possibilities to our fingertips and whims, practically anytime and anywhere. They're with us in our homes, our offices, our cars, on picnics, in the bathroom, and at ball games, just like coworkers, friends, and members of the family (except for in the bathroom). Computers and the Internet are now literal extensions of us. We take them for granted, well, like the sun.

I only wish adults had recognized from the outset that whenever we turn over an Internet connection to children we place in their hands one of the most powerful tools in the world. Have you heard the public service announcement that comes on at night right before the late local news: "It's 11 P.M. Do you know where your children are?" Imagine a child or adolescent, "safely" tucked away in his room at 11 P.M. with an electronic device and an Internet connection. "Where" could he be? The answer, potentially, is virtually anywhere in the world. The risk of being out late at night on the "digital" street corner, away from limits and boundaries of any kind, was (and still is) too abstract for many adults to foresee.

When it comes to kids and technology, I think we adults need to reframe the elephant: what an unsupervised Internet-ready device represents for a child is, in the starkest of terms, *unbridled independence*. And unbridled independence in any other form is something we would never turn over to a child, or even an unsupervised or insufficiently prepared adolescent. The mantra "Independence is earned" should come stamped on every device we bring into our homes.

I've saved this discussion for late in the book because too often the Internet is described as a "problem" in relation to kids. Not so. The Internet just is; it's not in itself a problem. What adults call problems—online predators, access to pornography, sexting, cyber bullying, posting unsavory images, the ungodly hours kids spend texting and networking, etc.—are merely symptoms and signs that from the beginning, adults let this one get right by us. (Maybe it was the gee-whiz factor.) The Internet is like the deep end of the pool, or driving on the interstate. Those aren't problems either. Letting kids play in it who can't swim well enough, or drive on it when they're novices, that would be a problem.

Nurturing children around something this powerful and diversified requires parents to wear their "suit," all five parts, literally for years. It will make a great wrap-up example in the next chapter.

Sex, Boundaries, and Intimacy

I played my first game of Spin the Bottle at a party when I was in sixth grade. It was great. Everyone had a turn and there was no pressure on anyone, since we were all friends and the game was based on chance. It was an exciting low-risk adventure, ideal for discovering what being close to someone in that way was like, if only for a second, without needing to "make the first move" or hazard a rejection. You kissed, or got kissed, because those were the rules. And since you always knew a parent could walk in at any moment, it felt perfectly safe, since nothing could get too far out of hand.

Kids *always* want to know the rules, and sex is no different, but there's another game most of us learn that's ultimately not so much fun. Do you remember "sexual" baseball, as in, going to "first," "second," or "third"? That's all about the rules, too, which explains its huge appeal and remarkable staying power in American culture, especially in third grade, when fourth or fifth graders will happily give you the entire playbook, from the first pitch to last.

You remember how it works, right? The batter (the boy) stares down the pitcher, with a determined look on his face: "Throw me anything—slow ball, fastball, curve, slider, no matter—I'm ready (for sex) at any time!" The boy gets to "score" if he can hit the ball far enough that he can trample the "bases" (in order: the girl's mouth, breasts, and genitals) and slide into "home" (OMG, her vagina!), while his teammates jump and cheer wildly at the bench. Since he only gets a point for going "all the way," the other bases—including oral or even anal sex in today's newer versions—really don't "count." (They're not *real* sex.) And if he "strikes out" and can't even get to "first," he's, well, a "loser," so he'll probably do or say anything to get there to maintain his bragging rights. (Or he'll just lie and say he did it anyway to avoid getting booed.)

Isn't that remarkable—the meaning of sex all laid out in a neat little package even a third grader can understand. (My sons were both in third grade when they first heard about "the bases," and so was I, a generation before; my students today, some well into high school, still speak this way.) Here's the problem, of course: baseball's a game, a competitive game, where someone has to lose so somebody else can win. Not only that, but in this particular game, one of the teams—the boys'—is always playing offense, and the other, the girls', only ever gets to play defense. Technically, in fact, the girls aren't really playing at all since they're the inanimate infield the game is played on. What kind of fun game is that?

And what an amazingly efficient model for transmitting to successive generations of third graders *everything* that's problematic about American sexual attitudes: for men, sex is about gamesmanship, ego-boosting, and social status, and for women, about objectification and cutting her losses. Since he's always on "ready" and expected to score (picture a batter's stance at the plate), if sex happens, it's going to be *her* fault for not defending her bases. But then again, if she doesn't let him "go far" enough, he'll find someone else. So which to invite: "slut" or "prude"? Pick your poison.

Could someone please call off the game?

Anyone under thirty reading this right now may be shaking his or her head and thinking I've got it all wrong. Things are different now, I am told all the time: The game today is equal, since the bases these days are often on the boy's body, too. I'll counter, however, that thinking of sex as sport—in any way (except good exercise)—is ultimately flawed. It invites exploitation and also precludes an understanding of sex as a form of intimacy based on trust and caring. Just because some girls might be playing "offense" now doesn't necessarily prove that anybody has been liberated from anything.

The only way to change things, as always, is for parents and teachers to make sure to get there first—well before the first pitch is called. Before kids ever hear or say the questions "How *far* should I go?" or "How *far* did you get?" we could in fact give them a whole different frame: sex is about closeness and intimacy, not "distance" and "getting." Indeed, where there's true intimacy, the line between giving and getting virtually disappears.

Intimacy and Boundaries

So, how can we best make the case?

Intimacy in *any* form is about blurring the boundaries between people. Probably the easiest kind of intimacy to understand is emotional intimacy. Much or most of the time we keep their deepest emotions to ourselves. Unless we're overwhelmed and can't keep our feelings in check, we usually pick with care the people with whom we share our deep personal selves. If you think about it, you could probably line up every piece of personal information that exists about you along a continuum, with the least personal at one end, let's say on the left, and the most personal at the end on the right. You are probably willing to share the information on the far left (what you do, city of birth, favorite sport, number of kids) with anyone, or practically anyone, but the pieces of information on the very far right you probably share only with the person or people you trust most in the world, if anyone. And you could likewise line up every other piece, in order, somewhere in between.

Most likely you could place all the people in your life along another line, too, with the ones you're least likely to tell your inner thoughts and feelings to whom on one end and those you trust the very most on the other. Or you could look at one particular relationship over the course of time in terms of how trusting you are of the other person and he or she of you. Where was your mother on the line when you were nine, thirteen, and eighteen, and if she is still alive, where would you place her now? Where would she put you?

Trust is powerful and dynamic, and a rich conversation topic with kids. Children and adolescents develop a natural and deepening understanding of the meaning of trust and intimacy as they mature. As soon as children begin to understand the idea of "best friend," as distinguished from "friend" and "good friend," they're well on the way. A best friend to a younger child is someone who's extra special, the friend you like being with the most, and someone you feel closer to than others. I think a wonderful time to introduce the concept of intimacy to children is whenever they become consciously aware of the feelings of closeness they have for other people, so that as early as possible "intimacy" and "closeness" can become part of their working vocabulary, like other household words. Parents could even talk to their infants about it—"Oh, it's so warm and intimate to snuggle and be close."

Older children and early adolescents develop a notion of intimacy based around the more abstract concept of trust, and at this stage, they almost always define trusting someone as "knowing they won't tell my secrets." It's good to help them think about trust and secrets in a broader way: "A friend not telling your secrets is a good *sign* of trust. People you can really trust have your best interests at heart and don't want to hurt you, and that's why they don't tell your secrets." That's a concept kids can really grow with, as you help them identify many other signs that tell you who can be trusted and under what circumstances, and who probably or definitely cannot.

As our kids move into adolescence, it's not uncommon for them to lose their sense of trust *in themselves*. How can you trust someone—even yourself—if you don't yet know who that person is, or is becoming, and you don't know what to expect? Their self-doubt can take a mighty, if temporary, toll on self-esteem; steady confirmation from us that *we* trust them, in all the many ways that we do, can help carry them through.

With greater confidence in their identity, older adolescents—often around age sixteen—become noticeably more "human." They begin to create increasingly authentic and less self-absorbed relationships, with peers and adults, and their closest relationships take on deeper textures and wider dimensions as they begin to think more like adults. Of course, the more deeply they trust, the more deeply they will feel betrayal, which is one reason romantic breakups can hit them so terribly hard.

Parents can deliberately create ongoing and overt life lessons about trust and intimacy from one developmental stage to the next, out of children's everyday experience. As with all abstractions, when we call concepts such as trust and intimacy by name, and show concretely how they work in everyday life, we make them relevant, useful, and real. And if we're aware and conscientious about connecting all the right dots, we can eventually turn these same conversations into a ready-made context for explaining the connections between trust, intimacy, boundaries, and sex.

Here's one approach I like quite a lot: Just as there are parts of our inner selves that are personal and not, there are parts of our bodies that we share freely with others—our face, hair, arms, shoulders—and some we keep private most of the time. As a relationship grows, and trust begins to emerge, two people may feel safe and confident enough to share deeper and deeper parts of their emotional selves. In a romantic relationship, they may want to share increasingly private areas of their physical and sexual selves, too—from holding hands, kissing, and touching faces, necks, arms, and legs, to touching breasts and genitals, to engaging in oral, anal, or vaginal intercourse. Where true intimacy exists, the physical and emotional sides of their relationship become mirror images of themselves. The line between giving and receiving begins to fade out, as each person takes more and more delight in the other person's pleasure, even more than their own.

That's a lot to process, and you would want to give it in steps, but an eleven-year-old student, hearing my sixth-grade version one day, caught the crux of it as nimbly as anyone I know, and explained it better, too: "I get it," he said. "When you think of it that way, you understand why sex can be special, or not. If you do certain things with everyone, those things just aren't special anymore. And if there's someone you really like, you can't let that person know how special they are *to you* unless you only do those things with them." Pretty amazing.

Changing the Language of the Conversation

Remember the bug zapper in the backyard that goes *bzzt* whenever an insect gets fried or anyone says the word "tweens" without putting quotes around it? Well, mine also goes off when I hear people say the word "sex" when they really mean "intercourse."

The sex = intercourse equation is a problem on many fronts. First of all, it confuses a category with an example, as if the United States were equal to

Maine. It's also blatantly heterosexist—since it effectively negates virtually every gay person in the world—and it ignores the variety and legitimacy of many other sexual experiences that all people can and do enjoy. But perhaps most problematic of all, the sex = intercourse definition of sex is essentially dehumanizing, since it reduces the experience of being sexual with another human being to the mere juxtaposition of parts. Where's the intimacy in that? By the way, the term "sexually active" is a big problem, too. Since it's usually a euphemism for intercourse, it creates all the same befuddling assumptions. Best to just say "intercourse" if that's what we mean.

When we talk in technicalities, rather than about meaning, we oversimplify and mislead. Many middle and high school kids I teach argue that a woman who has been raped has definitely "had sex." A penis and a vagina have touched, after all. What they're missing is that sex is to rape as sipping your favorite hot beverage is to having it poured down your throat.

If I had my druthers, we would all have our brains washed out so we could start over (and I could be done with all that racket in my brain). After all, the definition of sex *exclusively* as vaginal intercourse dates back many centuries, to a very different time and place when that was the *only* kind of sex permitted amoung some religious groups. Here's the kind of definition I would suggest for today's parents who want their children to value the sex/intimacy connection (eight's a good age to start): "I'm your go-to person about sex and I'm going to give it to you straight. Sex is a very special kind of intimacy or closeness. It's when two people hug, and kiss, and touch one another, and bring their bodies very close together, in ways that give their bodies wonderful feelings of pleasure, and under the best of all circumstances causes them to feel very close to each other."

Please note, there's purposefully no mention of body parts at all, or anyone's gender; the words are meant to be as inclusive as possible, and most of all, to communicate the *humanity* of being sexual with another human being. It's a definition meant to create plenty of space for giving information and guidance about sex going forward, all in the framework of intimacy. Telling young children that sex is about "love," as we often do, is a lovely sentiment that adults like to add, but not necessarily a connection young kids can meaningfully grasp. Love is an emotion, known to them only in limited ways that have virtually nothing to do with genital parts (except maybe loving the feelings they produce!). But physical intimacy they know, well, intimately, and have since you first held them in your arms.

Sex and Relationships?

I worry that the connection between sex and intimacy is a disappearing concept. When I first started teaching decades ago, sex and relationships were understood fundamentally as flip sides of each other, as two parts of an integrated whole. Make no mistake, many teens and adults at the time, as always, chose sex "just for sex," but they knew that separating the two was a clear departure from "standard." Gradually over the years, I heard an opposite set of assumptions take hold: Sex is sex. Relationships are relationships. And if you care to, you could *choose* to put them together. Today, for many young people in high school, college, and beyond—critical periods developmentally for learning the skills necessary for creating and sustaining intimate, long-term relationships—sex and relationships seem to operate in two fully separate spheres: Sex? Relationships? They go together?

Please don't misunderstand. I'm not making an appeal for the "good old days," which, of course, weren't always that good. But such fundamental changes over a relatively short period of time deserve our attention, and also candid conversation with our kids.

"Hooking up" is a phrase you'll definitely want to talk about because it's a perfect way in to all of these themes. But by all means, before you do, be sure to ask what *they* think the term means. To most adults I ask, "hooking up" is synonymous with depersonalized sex; two people who meet, often randomly, have a sexual experience, and then go their separate ways. (That's the way the media likes to define it, I think because it's yet another way to sensationalize teen sex and scare us to death.) But for teens, there is no standard definition; if you ask ten to fifteen kids, even in the same grade at the same school, you'll get at least six different meanings. When boys or girls say, "I hooked up with so and so," typically they mean, "We made out," which truly tells you nothing, since "making out," if you ask, can mean French kissing or intercourse or oral sex or anything and everything in between. So, unless you press for details, here's what you get: hooking up = making out, and making out = hooking up. With so much pressure on kids to get it sexually "just right"—with zero consensus about what that means—I'm convinced all this vagueness is a clever (and probably unconscious) ploy to keep their peers guessing and to avoid being judged.

Keep in mind—and here's another distinction—that the person they "hooked up" with, whatever they actually did, might have been a steady boyfriend or girlfriend, a friend (as in, "friends with benefits"), an acquaintance, or, indeed, a random person they met at a party with no intention of seeing again. All of these variables get lost unless we and they define our terms; when we do, "hooking up" is the perfect opening for helping kids sort out what specific behaviors are okay, or not, with whom, under what specific circumstances, and how best to decide. Be sure to parcel out the two separate issues that media sound bites almost always conflate: sex itself *and* the context in which it occurs. And use all of it to make clear *your* best advice and thinking about the relationship between sex and relationships.

Is Oral Sex Intimate?

Here's the quickest way to dispense with the tiresome argument over whether oral sex *is* sex: Like, duh, what's the second word in the phrase?

That done, how do we talk to our kids about what oral sex *means*? Thoroughly confused by the seemingly casual attitude toward oral sex among young people, so many adults say to me today, "When I was their age, oral sex was something way more intimate than intercourse, even. You had to *really* trust someone to even consider it. What gives?"

Though many people *still* blame Bill Clinton for this change in outlook, I have a very different take. When the story came out, the phrase "oral sex" was still in the closet. Most adults were simply unprepared to discuss the subject directly with their kids or even with other grown-ups. For months and months, truthfully, oral sex was the subject of endless jokes, silliness, and evasion. Many young people overhearing all this banter concluded, I'm convinced, that this was just not a topic or behavior to be taken particularly seriously. As always, it's us, not a fifty-year-old politician—even if he was at the time president of the United States—that kids look to for cues.

That said, and history aside, you know the drill: if you are a parent who wants your children to think of oral sex as an intimate behavior—and not "no big deal"—it's up to you to make the argument. Here's one of my favorites:

When you want to get to know people, you don't look at their feet. You look at their face. That's because people live in their faces. It's where you can see who they are, so faces are really personal. Faces are also where we keep all five of our senses: touch, taste, smell, sight, and hearing. So, here's the point: oral sex is a behavior where people put their face, truly the most personal part of their body, and where all five senses are located, right on top of someone else's sexual parts. Now that's an argument.

Back to Gender, Again

Nonrelational sex—sex with no intent or need for emotional intimacy or connection—is certainly not new under the sun. Over the centuries, though, the desire and ability to separate emotion from sex has been most often associated, at least stereotypically, with men. Women, as "they" used to say, have sex for love, while men have sex, well, for sex. There's a line in the movie *City Slickers* that sums up the sentiment best: "Women need a reason to have sex. Men just need a place."

To the extent that this was and is true, the reasons—biological, neurological, social, cultural, religious, political, and more—could fill another whole book. But what seems indisputable is that more girls and young women today are more publicly (and presumably privately) embracing a view where sex and emotions, let alone relationships, are easily compartmentalized (though as I've said before, I'm not sure that's as easily done as said; we take all of us wherever we go). Some people point to unhealthy cultural forces that surround girls today, and others say no, this is a sign of empowerment and the freedom, at last, to make the same choices as men. I'm certain that to some extent both views are true.

Regardless, I'm always suspicious when double standards rear their wily heads in not-so-obvious ways. Sex without attachment has been portrayed and accepted for men, accurately or not, as the norm for a very long time; how come, now that girls and women are "doing it," too, it's suddenly a problem? If emotion-free sex for girls is a worry, why haven't we been worried all along about boys and men, too? By the same token, it's girls in recent years who seem to be making all the change, away from the more traditionally female pattern to the more traditionally male. Real liberation doesn't happen without the freedom for both genders to make truly equal choices and to become more authentically themselves. I'll know that real and healthy change is afoot when I can walk through the halls on Monday mornings and over-hear a boy freely report to his friends, "Chris and I had such an amazing time Saturday night. We cuddled and kissed for hours." And I'll be especially pleased when gay kids feel just as free to share authentically about their weekends, too.

My own informal normative-belief research demonstrates, by the way, that both high school boys and girls, when surveyed anonymously, acknowl-edge they value sex (defined broadly) in the context of intimacy *highly*, girls only somewhat more so than boys. (Surprise, surprise: boys have feelings, too.) The biggest "a-ha" for my students is how wrong they were in predicting those results, especially in regard to the boys. They learn how deceiving the (loudest) sex talk they hear can be, and how it can silence kids who think they are different when they're really in the majority. I tell them all to stick with their gut, and never settle for anything less than what they really want. That's what I want for them most.

Some Final Thoughts

The world we live in today increasingly devalues privacy and basic respect for personal boundaries, to our great loss and even potential peril. Bound-aries are *fundamental* to our humanity, and to our right to be treated with respect. Objects, unlike people, have no boundaries and therefore have no rights; we can pretty much do with, and to, them as we please. All the atroc-ities committed in history have at their root the treatment of people as mere objects, not full human beings. To the degree that individuals or cultures ob-jectify people in any way, they become vulnerable to abuse.

On a personal level, when people disregard other people's boundaries, they take away a piece of them that should be theirs alone to give; when we disregard our own boundaries, we give away parts of us that rightfully should be earned by another person's trust.

Our personal boundaries hold us in and contain who we are. If we were to give away absolutely all of us to everyone, "we" would simply disappear. Holding on to our boundaries carefully is what makes it possible, ultimately, to create truly intimate relationships when we decide to let them go.

8

Anticipatory Guidance:
Turning Children
over to Themselves

For most of history, parents could reliably count on culture to reinforce the values and worldview they most wanted to pass on to their children. That was before mass media changed all of that, perhaps permanently. Today there are messages everywhere that contradict and potentially undermine many of parents' most cherished ideas about what constitutes a happy, healthy, and ethically correct life. Once it was hippies, flower children, and beatniks who were countercultural. Today there are parents who would feel very comfortable owning that label for themselves.[1]

Often I meet parents who lack confidence in what they believe. They say things like, "Well, I'm not really a prude, but the dancing kids do today really bothers me," or "Maybe I'm just old-fashioned, but I just don't think that kind of clothing is appropriate for twelve-year-olds." What they don't realize is that they've confused two very different things. Setting clear, age-appropriate limits around children's behavior has nothing at all to do with being uncomfortable or negative about sex, or about having outmoded values. It simply means you're doing your job as a parent and that you cherish and stand for important values, such as respect, privacy, and dignity. If those kinds of core values ever go out of fashion (and to a degree, haven't they?), we're really in trouble.

I was walking down the street in an upscale residential neighborhood on the West Coast a couple of years ago and passed by a children's clothing store. In the window was a display of Onesies, those blessed snap-on one-piece garments that infants wear. What made these stand out were the messages they sported: "I'm with MILF"; "Playground Pimp"; "Dad, get her a drink. She'll be nicer"; "Mother Sucker"; "Your Crib or Mine?"; "I only play with cute girls;" and a few others of this ilk. I'm one of those "If you see something, say something" kind of people, so I asked my husband to stay outside (he's one of those "Do I know her?" kind of people) while I went in to speak to the manager. I made a short speech about the harmful effects of sexualizing children and associating them with crude stereotypes and adult activities. She gave no reaction at all and barely looked up. *As soon as I leave,* I thought, *she's going to call me humorless and prudish, if not something worse.*

Talk about throwing out the baby with the bathwater! Where's the step-back, the ability to grasp that just because we supposedly don't see sex as "bad" anymore doesn't mean all uses of it are good?[2] It's another example of why I always put the words "so-called" in front of "sexual revolution." Here's where I think a piece of our culture got stuck in the post-'60s fallout, and where American popular culture most confuses and misleads: If oppression is always having to say no to things sexual, then liberation must mean *always saying yes.* Real liberation, of course, means the freedom *to make a real choice* based on terms that are on their own.

The ultimate purpose of nurturing is to oh-so-gradually turn our children over to themselves. In fact, just like the nurse in the pediatrician's office who charts their height and weight each year, we could just as easily track our children's journey toward independence and self-reliance by marking all the ways, big and small, they begin doing for themselves what we used to do *for* them. (My personal goal in this department: the day I no longer have to pay for my son's health insurance.) Though we may be ambivalent about this forward march away from us, we help them best by placing ourselves increasingly on the sidelines encouraging, supporting, cajoling, and—I'll admit to it—bribing them on.

Imagine if parents had the same philosophy about their children's emerging sexuality as they do, say, about preparing them to drive. The analogy isn't perfect, but there are many parallel lessons—about accountability, good judgment, assessing consequences, avoiding or at least minimizing risks, etc. But what really interests me is where the analogy most fundamentally breaks down.

Most grown-ups accept as a matter of fact that young people *will* drive, will *want* to drive, will *enjoy* driving, and most likely will *need* to drive to function well as independent adults. These expectations are "in the air" and out in the open long before kids ever apply for a permit or turn on the ignition. Even when children are young, parents and other adults don't hesitate for a second to teach them a thing or two about driving—whenever it occurs to them—because everyone acknowledges that driving is a part of life that someday will be part of kids' lives, too. Long before teenagers actually get out there on the road, their world is set up to support them in managing this part of their independence, eventually, as well as they possibly can.

Here's another way to put it: When it comes to driving, from the get-go we educate children for "yes," as in, "YES, you will almost certainly drive someday, and we'll help you get it right." But when it comes to their sexuality, we most often take the opposite tack: We don't educate for yes, but for no, or "not yet." We're afraid to say, "YES, you will almost certainly engage in sexual behaviors in your life, and we'll help you get it right." Starting out with a negative about sex may *feel* less risky and more protective, but really, why should it? Driving a car is potentially more dangerous than almost any kind of sex, and besides, we certainly don't hesitate to talk about driving with a six- or ten- or fourteen-year-old for fear she'll take the minivan out for a spin.

Remarkably, despite sweeping changes in how children and adolescents live, Americans still embrace paradigms suited for a far distant past. Before the twentieth century, young people were considered adults by the time they were sixteen. That's when many boys completed their apprenticeships or took their place as adult workers on the family farm. Sixteen was also the average age when girls first got their periods and when many commonly got married. It was a simpler time for young people developmentally, since physical, sexual, social, and vocational maturity peaked for most young people at about the same age. Today we are much less certain about when exactly adulthood begins. High school graduation? Military service? Full-time job? Starting college? Voting age? Graduate school? Financial independence? Cohabitating? Marriage? (Paying for your own health insurance?) Who the heck knows?

One thing is certain: With the average age of heterosexual marriage now twenty-six for women and twenty-eight for men (and even higher for college-educated adults), and the average age of reproductive capacity for girls now twelve and a half, and thirteen and a half for boys, young people today (and their parents) face an unprecedented challenge: how to manage a thirteen-to fourteen-year gap between sexual and reproductive maturity and marriage. Even the phrase "premarital sex" seems anachronistic in today's world: When would the "premarital" period actually begin? And hold on to your hats and your pocketbooks, ladies and gentlemen: some experts are now identifying yet a new developmental stage, what they call "second adolescence" or the "odyssey years," during which young adults continue to explore their options and identities.[3] If thirty is indeed the new twenty, it will mean that an increasing number of very late twenty-somethings will only just then be coming into full adulthood. Even the Merriam-Webster dictionary confirms it! One of its newly added entries is "boomerang child," a designation for adult children who leave home, only to return later on in their twenties during this additional exploratory stage. (Returning home is also a sign of the times economically.)

Clearly it's time for a change in our thinking. Parents (and society at large, but don't count on that terribly soon) need to reconsider the way we prepare children to manage their sexuality during an ever-expanding developmental stage. What they sorely need is a middle ground between an "always say yes" popular culture and the official adult position of educating for no, or "not yet." We simply can't empower them to make good choices, which inevitably they will need to make, if we continue to act as if their only good option is "don't." When the time comes to make a decision, how will they know how to choose?

Educating for Yes

Educating for yes, not for no or "not yet," could sound something like this: "Children, sex will most likely be a part of your life, starting perhaps in middle school, and it's our job as your parents, as always, to help you manage this part of you, too." (Oops, did you just read "sex" as "intercourse"? It's a very hard habit to break.) See how much less scary that sentence feels now that sex could mean, say, French kissing?

Educating for yes is based on the premise that sex is not the same thing as vaginal intercourse, but a range of behaviors along a continuum of increasingly intimate behaviors. A "sexual experience" in the eighth grade may be very far removed from intercourse in any form, but it requires anticipatory guidance from parents *no less*. Indeed, these early experiences, in whatever form they happen to take, can be powerful both in the moment and for the future. Whether good, bad, or indifferent, they can set patterns in motion with far-reaching impact on emotions, relationships, expectations, communication, boundaries, integrity, self-esteem, self-agency, and gender roles.

Remember, too, that since educating for yes is a form of anticipatory guidance, it's only one of the five roles parents need to constantly play. It will be helpful only if we keep building the foundation, by knowing who our children are and what behaviors they can and can't manage; teaching them about their bodies, their own development, and physical, social, and emotional risks; naming the values we expect them to bring to all situations in life, with sex no exception; and by providing adequate supervision around their social lives so they don't end up out of our range with more rope and opportunity than they can handle.

The Experience of "Being Sexual"

Remember, it's *the experience of being sexual with another person* that's the issue (not the particular juxtaposition of parts). I'd love Merriam-Webster to give us a new word for that phenomenon, too. One of my students suggested the verb "sexing" (not to be confused with the media-coined term "sexting"), which the rest of the class found sort of clever. After all, we call walking "walking" and speaking "speaking," not "having forward motion" or "having speech." What does it mean, really, to "have" sex? It's not exactly something you put in your pocketbook or wallet or into a drawer. Once again, it's the ancient Hebrews, perhaps, who may have gotten it right. In the Old Testament, the word for "sex" is a verb—*lada'at*—that also means "to know."

I'm reminded of a story that still touches my heart. A young man, a rising high school senior, came to talk to me, as he had from time to time over the previous two years. When he was a sophomore in high school, his parents—family friends—designated me as a consultant, an adult outside the family he might go to for help or support about certain things he might wish to keep private. (A smart idea—if you're comfortable with it—and there's someone you trust.) The question this time was, "How will Maggie and I know when we're ready to have sex?"

I said something next that at first took him aback. "Will, I don't mean to pry or make you uncomfortable, but I would have assumed that you and Maggie are *already* having sex." "Huh?" the look on his face plainly said. "No, here's what I mean. You and Maggie have had a wonderful relationship for almost two years. Lots of adults, even, envy the way the two of you communicate. You're both very affectionate, you obviously care about each other very deeply, and I know you spend time alone. When I said 'sex,' I didn't mean intercourse. I meant that I assumed you and Maggie are having a sexual relationship of *some kind*. It might be kissing, for all that I know, and besides, the particulars are none of my business. But whatever kind of physical relationship it happens to be, I also assume it's pretty wonderful because of the emotional relationship the two of you share."

Will's face broke out into a very wide grin. "In fact," I said, "my guess is you're probably having a *way more* wonderful experience than some of your friends or peers who might be having intercourse." "You're right," he said. "I am having sex. In fact, I'm having wonderful sex! More wonderful sex than a lot of my friends!" (He had clearly given up the idea of feeling deprived.) "Now I know what to do. Maggie and I need to talk about what's different about intercourse and other things we've been doing, and whether we're ready for *that*."

Once sex wasn't officially only *one* particular act, he was able to discover on his own the right questions to ask and consider.

Make no mistake, educating for yes doesn't mean your kids will actually *say yes* to any particular sexual experience: it means teaching them how to think clearly about both yes and no *as options*. Educating for no or "not yet," ironically much like the message "anything goes," offers a point of view, but not a way of arriving at one. What kids need most, as they go on to navigate years and years of yes/no decisions, are tools for evaluating when it might be okay to say yes; when it's more prudent to say no; and when it's time to say, "I've got to think about this some more"—*no matter the specific behavior.* Even those young people who choose to say no to *all* sexual experiences until they are married still need education for yes. How else will they know what they are waiting for, or how to create a healthy and satisfying sexual life when the time comes?

Something else to consider is this: When we give our kids direct permission to say no *or* yes to sexual experiences we think are appropriate for their age, we probably increase the chances they'll more thoughtfully consider saying no. Almost all people—adults and kids—make more deliberate decisions when they're taught how to think about them, and the process typically slows things down since they become more selective. Also, it puts the responsibility for sexual decisions much more squarely on kids' shoulders, which is where it ultimately belongs; the more responsibility we ask them to take for their own choices and their outcomes, the more they'll learn how to make decisions on their own terms, because they'll discover what those terms are.

Many adolescents passively "let things happen" in sexual situations, often because they don't know their "terms" ahead of time and/or can't find their voice. Others drink their way into sexual experiences, precisely so they won't have to make fully conscious choices, and then, in a form of double-dip denial, rationalize their behavior later with an "alcohol made me do it" defense. There are legions of factors, societal and developmental, that impede sexual accountability among teens, and just as many that fuel underage alcohol use and abuse. It's no wonder alcohol and sex are such not-so-strange bedfellows, and with such potentially dangerous consequences. All the more reason, I would argue, for parents to equip their kids, very deliberately, with the self-knowledge and confidence to deal forthrightly with sexual choices.

Back to Gender

Especially for heterosexual teens, there are almost always powerful gender dynamics at work. Girls in the United States, raised on "sexual baseball," understand on some level that the rules of sex are rigged, and not in their favor. So long as they agree to play out their assigned roles, they are essentially doomed to second-class citizenship, where no matter their choices, they will be open to the kinds of judgments that boys are not. Some girls decide the way out and up is to "play like a boy." I hear from many parents that the tables are turned today, that it's their sons who are under pressure by girls pursuing *them* for sexual experiences. I wonder whether girls who choose to go down this path have asked themselves first, "What would it look like, actually, to 'play like a girl'?" If girls (and boys) were to make up new rules for themselves that were a win-win for everybody, what would they be?

Girls who internalize their second-class status, and don't know they've done it, are the ones who concern me the most. The sexual double standard implies that girls and women are inferior and don't deserve better. Many girls put up with sexual mistreatment—harassing behaviors, disrespect for their boundaries, expectations for "servicing," disregard for their pleasure or desires—because deep down inside they're conditioned to think that's just the way it is, or worse, it's what they deserve or all they can expect. Most worrisome of all, many don't recognize what they experience *as* mistreatment, or if they do, dismiss it as "just boys being boys."

Paradoxically, some girls, previously belittled by callously unfair rumors or taunts, try to regain control by deliberately inviting similar slurs, even acting as if they relish the idea; at least, they think, they've brought the negative attention on themselves, rather than waiting to become a victim. What a terribly sad way to cope. They also may discover a gratifying but false sense of power in controlling access to something certain boys want. Often these girls will need help to restore their inner sense of confidence and worth, and to embrace healthier ways of coping with the vicissitudes of adolescence and discovering what it is they want for *themselves*.

I am always most surprised by girls who in every other way are really free thinkers, but when it comes to sexuality seem to blindly follow a script. One particularly independent-minded tenth grader told me about going to a party where she met a guy, whom she described as "okay," who wanted to have intercourse. She said she wasn't interested and he asked her to give him a blow job instead. And she did. She told me all of this nonchalantly as part of a longer story, which was why she came to talk in the first place. Eventually I went back to the part about her and the guy and said I was curious about why she had gone along. That one simple question just blew her away. "Oh my God," she said. "Why did I do that? I didn't even think about it."

The girls I know who make the healthiest decisions are those who actively and thoughtfully take ownership of their sexual selves. They are amazingly powerful. They know in advance what they will do and won't, and why, and under what circumstances, and they communicate their boundaries, and their sexual needs and desires, openly and clearly. They expect to be treated with respect, and recognize and refuse to buy into anything less. If they need to use physical protection, they come prepared. They have respect for others and their right to make their own choices without pressure or coercion. They're not habitual "pleasers," as girls often feel they must be, and they can say "thanks, but no thanks" without feeling guilty or obliged. Not surprisingly, they are in the minority, and also way more likely to be older teens than young ones, and to have parents who are decidedly hands-on.

One of the best gifts parents can give their daughters is precisely the kind of sexual "self-agency" that is at the very heart of educating them for yes. When we give girls overt permission to choose yes in situations we think are appropriate and healthy for their age, it puts *them* psychologically in charge of their decisions, yes or no. This gift—the freedom to take responsibility for their own choices—is how we can help them become equal, not second-class. For girls, starting when they are thirteen or fourteen, it's the modern-day version of "the talk." We can ask: What do *you* really want *just for yourself* in relationships? How do you *want* to be treated? What are or will be *your* conditions for saying yes to any particular sexual experience? I can't count the number of therapists who've told me they treat young women, from their teens to their late twenties, who don't know how to begin to answer let alone to ask themselves these questions.

Contrary to the stereotype of boys' sexual self-confidence and swagger, boys need support and permission to make decisions on their own terms, too. It's always very revealing when the subject of male rape comes up in my class; most boys are incredulous that such a thing could actually happen. Many boys laugh because they're plainly uncomfortable, but others laugh because they honestly find the whole idea, well, laughable. No man, they argue, would turn down sex if it were available, so in addition to men's relative strength, how could a man possibly be raped? (They also can't imagine a woman ever needing to "pay" a man for sex, since he would usually just jump at the chance.) To them, sex for a man is always a no-brainer: Where's the thoughtfulness or self-agency in that?

Once a year or so a high school boy comes to see me, feeling devastated. The stories are very similar. Each time, the boy has been in a situation where a girl made it clear that she wanted to have intercourse. At the time, he wasn't sure it was what *he* wanted, but felt he had to go along. His body, however, knew himself better than he did, and refused to participate. Unable to keep his erection, he had been totally mortified. (Mercifully, in almost every instance, the girl was kind and understanding.) By the time he gets to my office, he's feeling horrible about himself, and convinced there must be something terribly wrong with him.

My goal each time is to walk boys through the assumptions that made them feel as if they had only *one* choice. (I also reassure them there's not a male on the planet whose penis cooperates each and every time.) I ask them, too, what they really wanted to do in the situation they were in. Some say they're not sure; others acknowledge they wished they could just kiss, touch, and cuddle. In the most recent case, the boy resolved to make another date and say, "Here's what I really want to do, and that's just to be physical with you in a low-key way so we can get to know each other slowly."

For me, these talks are always a reminder of how much external and internal pressure boys are under to want sex in any form, grab it at any time and every opportunity, and "perform" it flawlessly. To find their own terms, most boys need two things from the adults in their lives: reminders that they are entitled to have choices, and ongoing support for recognizing and resisting anyone's assumptions to the contrary, including their own. Keep your eyes and ears wide open for references to "boys will be boys" thinking and expectations—you'll find they're embedded and spoken outright everywhere in American culture. Tell your kids, starting when they're as young as seven, what you think about the stereotypes these references expose. Get mad, and show it, whenever boys and men are depicted disrespectfully. Eventually you'll be able to connect the dots to stereotypical sexual expectations, too.

Ask, Don't Tell

When people ask me, "What do you teach?" I'm tempted to answer, "Hopefully, critical thinking." Whenever you help your children work through a problem, or evaluate their options, or see something in a different way, that's exactly what you teach, too. One of the best ways to help our kids navigate sexual decisions, now and into the future, is to teach them not what to think, but *how*.

Asking questions that promote thoughtful reasoning is a skill in itself. The kinds of questions that make people think are open-ended; they don't point to a definite right or wrong answer, but are intended to generate lots of *possible* answers. Also, they are crafted to prompt sentence- or paragraph-long responses, not a simple yes or no. In contrast, "leading" questions—for example, "Don't you think sixteen is too young to have an exclusive boyfriend?"—are stacked; the supposed right answer is offered within the question itself. (In fact, leading "questions" are really statements in disguise: "Here's what I think. You agree with me, right?") The purpose of open-ended questions is not to pry, or to get information, or to get someone around to your point of view. They are for the benefit of the person being asked, not the person doing the asking.

Here's a host of questions to sharpen your children's reasoning skills about sexual decisions before they need to make them, and/or whenever their social life seems to shift into a higher gear. They help bring clarity to issues that most thirteen- to eighteen-year-olds think about and spiral back to again and again on deeper levels as they move through their teenage years. Notice especially the topics that might be hard for you to listen to or discuss in an objective way—where you would want to jump in with your opinion and tell your son or daughter *what* to think, not *how*. The questions aren't intended at all as a script; you know your kids best, and you'll want to phrase your questions in ways that are a good fit for them. I offer them as suggestions—you'll think of more (and better) ones as you go along. And of course, you'll want to add your opinions, after you've listened carefully to your kids'.

When you're (inevitably) having trouble holding your tongue, here's the thing to keep in mind: the more you show genuine interest and respect in what your children have to say, the more they'll want to hear you out, too—if not today, then at some other time. Also, even if their ideas right now are simplistic or shortsighted, it's really no cause for alarm. If you're keeping tabs and setting the right limits, they won't be making decisions anytime soon that are out of their range. Encouraging critical thinking and reflection doesn't preclude or substitute at all for age-appropriate limit-setting, so that no matter how "smart" they are, or think they are, their choices and behavior remain well within parameters they are ready to handle.

Remember, too, that your children are a work in progress, and never a finished product. Even if you're unimpressed or disappointed by their conclusions or how they reach them, give it another week or month or year. They will grow, and your questions, your sincerity, and your patience will help move them along. Above all, keep doing a "tone check" on yourself and your "agenda." What almost always works is an approach that's sincerely invitational—you can use things that naturally come up around you, or frame it as a curiosity that just popped into your head—and collegial, where your goal is "wondering out loud" *with* your child in the spirit of inquiry. In fact, try to identify conversations in the past about another topic altogether where you and your child have enjoyed being in that kind of mode with each other, and try for *that* tone. And remember, don't confuse "talking" with "doing"; your child will not think that because you're raising stuff it means you're worried he's doing stuff or that you think he should.

- What sexual behaviors do some of your friends think are okay for your age and not? Do you agree or not? Why? Do you know whether they enjoy those experiences, both boys and girls? Do kids talk about what they do sexually in a public way? How do you feel about that? Do you think they tell the truth or not? How do you know?
- In what ways do boys' and girls' attitudes seem alike and different? Are boys and girls judged in different ways because of what they do sexually? What are your thoughts on that? Are they judged if they are gay? Do boys ever do sexual things they're not sure they want to do? Girls? Why do you think that happens? What do you think

would be comfortable sexually for you at your age? How about next year, or the year after? What would be some good ways to handle it if you and another person didn't agree about what you were comfortable with? What might be hard about the situation?

✓ What are reasons and motivations young people have for being sexual? How often, do you think, are their reasons really *non*sexual—for example, to seem more grown-up, to hold on to a boyfriend or girlfriend, to impress their friends or peers, to please someone else, or to prove something about themselves? What reasons do you think are the right ones?

✓ Do kids ever talk about "hooking up" or "friends with benefits" or "bases"? How would they define what these mean? What are some advantages or disadvantages of thinking about sex in those ways? Which ones make most sense to you? How well should people know and care for each other when they share sexual experiences?

✓ Have you ever been in a situation where you thought you were ready to do something new and it turned out you weren't? What information was missing that led you to make the wrong call? What did you learn? Did you learn anything about yourself? How does a person know whether he or she is ready for a certain sexual experience? What questions does she need to ask herself? How do you find out—for sure—whether the *other* person is ready, too, or if the relationship is ready for that kind of intimacy? How can both people best check out their motivations?

A final note about being "ready." When I ask kids how they would know if they were ready for a sexual experience, they most often say, "Oh, you just know in your gut." Not so, I tell them. There may be too much at stake. This kind of knowing is not in your gut—it's in your head. "Ready" is about knowing the right questions to ask yourself, and being honest about the answers. If you think it's about your gut, or can't think of any questions, or can't be honest with yourself, you're not ready, or at the very least you're not prepared. I remind them, too, that "ready" even under the best of circumstances is never a sure thing. That's the point of new experiences: you don't really know what can or will happen until you get there. The best you can do is to deliberate beforehand as carefully as you can.

As parents, how do we know our children are ready, especially for sexual behaviors that carry significant risk? There's no magical yardstick for sexual readiness that's different from any other kind: readiness is as readiness does. How careful and thoughtful are your kids right now? How well do they plan ahead? How well do they handle their responsibilities, their relationships, and their emotions? How self-reliant are they? What are their core values? How much responsibility do they take for their physical health, and how well do they respect and care for their bodies? What do they know about protection, both physical and emotional? How well do they know themselves? How vulnerable are they to manipulation by others, or to manipulating them? How assertively do they communicate, and how easily do they read others' motivations and needs? To what degree can they put the needs and wishes of other people first? How much respect do they show for boys, for girls, and for sex itself?

Measuring their capacities for these benchmarks in their lives overall will give you a good sense of the kinds of sexual experiences they might be ready for and not.

Gay and Trans Kids

In the book I wrote for parents and educators more than a decade ago, *Sex and Sensibility,* there is a separate chapter on kids who are gay or transgender. I wanted to shine a spotlight on the mistreatment they suffered and the lack of available support in many of their communities, and to make a plea for adults everywhere to make change happen.

It's a decade later, and change *has* happened. The best barometer I have is the youth summit sponsored every two years for LGBTQ kids—lesbian, gay, bisexual, transgender, and questioning—by our local chapter of the Gay, Lesbian, and Straight Education Network (GLSEN). Years ago the young people who attended came from a handful of regional high schools, public and private. There was little diversity among them racially, ethnically, geographically, or socioeconomically. The kids themselves appeared reserved and tentative, even a little afraid, and they hung back in discussion. They had very little basic information about LGBTQ issues, their right to go to school in a safe environment, or resources available to them. Most were not involved in any kind of advocacy work, and they were ill informed about relevant current events and their legal and political implications for the LGBTQ community.

Today the kids who attend the conference are anything but shy. They are remarkably diverse, connected, energized, excited, and articulate. They are mobilized, organized, political, and impressively well educated about "their" issues. Many are "out" at home and more open at school (the number of GSAs, or Gay Straight Alliance clubs, in US schools quadrupled from 2001 to 2008).[4] And most important, they are proud. What I see in these kids, compared to those years ago, is that they feel affirmed. The affirmation may not be consistent or exist in every domain, but there are now places, role models, events, dialogue, and media that affirm the existence and value of gay kids.[5] As I've said, affirmation—for gay kids, as all kids—is need number one because it's need number one.

Beyond support and affirmation—along all of its dimensions—what LGBTQ kids need from their parents is mostly the same, too. Practically everything in this book applies directly to kids who are sexually "different." The same core needs always apply; kids who are LGBTQ just may need *extra layers* of information, clarity about values, limit-setting, and/or anticipatory guidance.[6] And because they are "different" (in this one particular way) from the average or the expected, and often live and grow up in environments where there is ignorance and insensitivity—if not outright intolerance and hostility—most will need extra help anticipating and coping with additional stressors and hardships in what is already a challenging period developmentally.

For many LGBTQ kids, things have not changed nearly enough. In one recent national survey, 84.6 percent reported being verbally harassed, 40.1 percent reported physical harassment, and 19 percent reported being physically assaulted at school. Like all students who are repeatedly harassed for being "atypical," these young people are at significantly higher risk for depression, substance use, absence and withdrawal from school and school-related activities, academic failure, and suicide. By far, the young people most at risk are those who experience rejection at home, especially those who are tossed out or who find the situation so devastatingly hurtful they feel they must leave. Many end up homeless and fending for themselves on the street.

In the wake of high-profile news reports highlighting suicides and other tragedies among LGBTQ youth, it's vital to remember that many, many gay youth lead productive, healthy, and happy lives, and increasingly so. All gay kids and their parents need to focus on this reality, even when their individual situations at present are fraught with difficulty; it's an especially important message for the 10 percent to 15 percent of gay kids who are thought to be emotionally fragile and at risk for serious physical and mental health problems, such as alcohol and other drugs use and depression. The picture today is more difficult and complex for trans children and teens, even those who have supportive families, but their issues are beginning to receive much more positive attention in the press and television news. With greater familiarity and education will come greater understanding and acceptance of the reality that some children and teens legitimately need and want to express themselves in ways that do not match their biological gender according to traditional role expectations.

When parents discover that their child is "different" in these ways, or in any other significant way than they thought, it can present difficult challenges.[7] We all have ideas, fantasies, dreams, and expectations that revolve around who we think our children are, or who we need and want them to be, and what and who they will become. Adjusting to the reality that our children's lives do not and will not match up with some of our hopes and expectations can feel like a blow, and we need to give ourselves the gift of time and space to adjust and let go of what might have been. (The more we can do of this in private, the better, lest our children misinterpret the letting-go process as a rejection of them and their identity.) On the other side of that process will be the discovery that our children, in every other way, are exactly who they have always been and are meant to be. In time, you will have new dreams for them, and for you. In the meantime, starting from the day you know, they will need your love for them to be stronger than any pain or upset you may experience.

Many parents adapting to these new realities also benefit from education and *re*-education about the nature of gender and sexual diversity. Understanding, for example, that parents don't "make" their kids gay or transgender, any more than they can "make" their kids straight or gender congruent, can dispel outdated and guilt-inducing "scientific" theories, often the product of biased research. They'll discover the prevailing view today is that gay "just is," not the product of something "gone wrong." And they'll get a reality check on negative and misleading stereotypes that portray the LGBT individuals and their lives as inherently and globally "different"—as "them," not "us." As my friend Marla likes to say about her lesbian-headed family, "The reality of our lives is really *not* very different at all. I'm partnered to a doctor, we have a teenage daughter, two dogs, live in a house in the country, and drive a Volvo station wagon. What part of the 'all-American dream' is missing? What's truly different is the stigma, rejection, and discrimination we and our child face."

Kids who are LGBTQ, too, need reality testing and exposure to the huge diversity of young people and adults who compose their community, and also to straight and non-trans "allies" who can offer a whole other layer of acceptance and affirmation. Local groups in many cities, counties, and states provide excellent counseling, educational programs and materials, and support groups for both young people and their families. Many organizations also offer young people (and their parents) vital opportunities for interacting with happy, well-adjusted, and successful LGBT adults, and for all-important age-appropriate socialization in safe and supervised spaces with their LGBTQ peers. National organizations such as PFLAG (Parents and Friends of Lesbians and Gays) and GLSEN (Gay, Lesbian, Straight Education Network) can help you find resources in your area. Both of their websites—and others listed in the family resource list at the end of this book—provide legions of useful information for parents, kids, and educators.

Those "Extra Layers" of Anticipatory Guidance

As we know, the developmental "tasks" of adolescence are formidable, to say the least. It's a time for consolidating your identity; separating gradually from parents; identifying with and looking for support and validation increasingly from peers versus family; gaining independence; and learning how to integrate sexuality and romance into your life in positive and healthy ways. And did I mention planning your future, and figuring out how to pay for your own health insurance? *Wow!*

Many of these challenges can be immeasurably more complex for LGBTQ preteens and teens, and as a consequence they require extra doses of anticipatory guidance from caring and tuned-in adults.[8] The tragic implications for young people who, for emotional and/or practical reasons, feel they must remain closeted at home, school, places of worship, and elsewhere are clear: they must essentially *raise themselves* around many important developmental milestones, while coping on their own, silently and invisibly, with a hostile and sometimes hateful and even physically dangerous environment.

For kids who are out to close friends and supportive adults—especially their parents and family—their needs are relatively straightforward. First of all, they need space, time, and permission to grow into their own unique sexual and gender identity (along the sexual and gender continua described in Chapter 5), without the pressure to self-label, or being labeled by others, prematurely. They, and their parents, may need extra help and support, too, if they're connected to a cherished ethnic or religious group, or an extended family, that holds inflexibly negative judgments about sexual or gender diversity.

LGBTQ kids also need adults to teach them coping skills for dealing with the rejection, ridicule, or harassment they may encounter, and who will step up to the plate in situations, such as chronic bullying at school, that they are powerless to stop on their own. Their physical and emotional safety must always come first. There are many terrific resources to help schools create socially, emotionally, and physically safer environments for LGBTQ kids,[9] and that will mean safer environments for *all* kids: in a school where any one group is singled out for mistreatment and the mistreatment is allowed to continue, kids know their identity group could well be next. Moreover, since a large percentage of straight kids now know and often feel close to people who are LGBTQ, whenever gay or trans students are treated cruelly, they, too, often suffer in silence. They may also feel they must cling to rigid gender-role stereotypes that don't fit who they truly are either, for fear that they may become the next target of bullying or harassment.

Apart from all that, what kids who are LGBTQ need—provided for them very directly and deliberately—is what *all* teens need, and you know the drill: factual *information* about their bodies and development, about STIs, sexual

assault, and pregnancy prevention (many will at some point engage in heterosexual intercourse), and about the dangers of mixing sexual decisions and behavior with alcohol and other drugs; support for developing their personal
values connected to sex and relationships; expectations around respecting their
own and others' sexual *boundaries*; and *guidance* about venturing into intimacy, dating, and relationships. As with straight kids, remember that it's not
about "sex," but rather nurturing healthy sexuality, with extra attention paid to
their unique needs and circumstances. Here's a clear example a high school
student pointed out: "What do I do if my boyfriend isn't out to his parents, but
my parents have a rule for me and my siblings that they have to meet the parents of people I date?" Gay kids, and their parents, often can't just take for
granted many of the things others can: straight kids and adults are always "out."

It helps put things in perspective, too, to remember that gay and trans kids
are just kids, struggling, all of them, with some of the most universal and
human questions of all: Am I attractive? Likeable? Loveable? Will anyone
ever like me as more than a friend? How will I know? How can I meet new
people? How much intimacy am I ready for? Do I smell okay? What's the best
way to ask someone out? Could I be gay? What do you do on a first date?
Who kisses whom first? Open mouth, or not? What do you do next? How do
you *not* make a fool of yourself? What if you have to pee? How do you say
no? When do you say yes? What's the best way to break up? How can I deal
with my hurt? How do you know if you're really in love?

We can *all* relate, can't we?

Technology: Keeping One Hand on the Wheel

Our children's independence just happens. They are internally programmed
for growth and development, and in most ways they just take us along for
the ride. There are times, though, when we need to take control of the keys,
the headlights, the brakes, and even the map. (Even then, they're always in the
driver's seat.) Technology, for example, is so powerful and pervasive in children's lives we need to sit right up front in the passenger seat until they can
at least *think* like adults.

A colleague told me a story about meeting a girl who was in the second
grade. "Will you be my friend?" the girl asked. Then she asked for the

woman's e-mail address. The woman was confused until she realized the girl was asking her, a total stranger, to be her Facebook "friend."

Social networking is, well, very friendly. It's an absolutely brilliant idea that has changed millions of lives in countless positive ways.[10] (It has also made a lot of other people very wealthy. Though people, especially children and teens, think of social networking as free, there are potentially huge costs to users in terms of privacy loss, constant targeting and sharing of information about them by marketers, and the amassing of limitless information about their personal habits and interests chronicled from childhood.)[11] But, like everything else on the Internet, social networking is not a toy and it's definitely not benign. In the hands of a child or a teenager (and even many adults), it can be a disaster.

A major reason that adults take too much of a hands-off approach regarding their children's use of technology—astonishingly, only a little more than three in ten young people report their parents put limits on their use of the computer—is that they feel inadequate. "My kids know way more than I do about computers," they lament. "I don't even know where to start. Why would they listen to me?" What parents forget, points out David Delmonico, an expert on kids and technology at Duquesne, is that although their children may have a higher TQ (technology intelligence quotient), parents have a much higher EQ (emotional intelligence quotient). In other words, they have the real-world experience and the intellectual, social, and emotional maturity to imagine, and safely manage, the *power* of the Internet, even if they are far from being experts on the technology itself.

Delmonico says that young people online perceive themselves to be in a comfortable "safe zone." With the computer located usually in a physically protected and familiar environment, they feel isolated, insulated, and anonymous. Also, the online world has a fantasy-like quality to it that makes it seem as if the everyday rules of life—such as no lying, or cheating, or being mean—don't apply. (Kids need to know that right and wrong are exactly the same on the Internet as in "real" life.) If something ever happens online that feels upsetting or scary, they can just push "escape" and make it all vanish— but not really, since the Internet "never forgets." What's more, interactive online experiences have an equalizing effect, since everyone in communication, no matter the age or true identity, is simply "chatting" or "friending" or bonding over like interests or needs.

Of course, messages sent online or via cell phone or text are probably the least secure form of communication in the world.[12] Kids are often stunned when "caught" sending, receiving, or posting compromising information or images, and may even feel violated that someone has dared invade their "privacy." The problem is they can't see far enough beyond their computer or cell phone screen to imagine the great big world on the other side.

Parents and other adults would do well first to understand and affirm their adolescents' wild (and sometimes wooly) love affair with technology and the Internet. Both provide an unparalleled vehicle—and a parallel universe—for them to try on new identities, stay in *constant* touch with friends and peers, and get *immediate* feedback, support, and advice. What's more, they get to create their own "real-life" dramas, in front of a virtual audience of their peers, and also to chronicle their entire adolescence for posterity in images, writing, and song. And in the process, they get to take risks, practice independence, explore separation from parents, and learn more things about more things in the universe than anyone ever could have imagined. I have a feeling that Erik Erikson, one of the first psychologists to describe the psychosocial stages of adolescence, would be blown away by such a perfect developmental match.

Multiply all this power, independence, and opportunity by a factor of dozens, or even hundreds, of kids in constant communication with one another, and, well, you get the picture. By not minding the computer store, or the Internet connections at home, we've allowed kids to create a monster of potential misuse and abuse right alongside of, and entwined with, extraordinary opportunities for healthy and positive learning and growth. Many kids send dozens, if not scores, of texts to their friends before they even leave for school; they sleep with their cell phones and laptops; they watch (and sometimes make) pornography in the middle of the night; they spend an average of seven hours in front of their multiple screens, not doing homework, every single day; they stream their escapades live; they trust friends with nude photos of themselves, only to hear they've gone viral one morning as they walk into school; they give away personal information to strangers in chat rooms and on networking sites; they participate in cyber bullying; they post compromising images of themselves online that will be scrutinized by prospective admissions officers and employers—all, well, simply because they can.

A few years ago, a third-grade teacher told me she'd just taken a cell phone away from a boy on the playground who'd used it to take a photo up a girl's skirt. "Just wait," she said. "This is only the beginning." If only all of us had been as clairvoyant about the powerful devices on the horizon—developed and designed for *adult* use, let's remember—and how dramatically they would also change the lives of our children and teens. And speaking of cell phones, the idea of a third grader owning a cell phone would have been considered utterly outrageous ten years ago. (My son graduated from college in 2002 and he and his friends didn't own or even want one!) What did we think or know about the nature of third graders a decade ago, I always ask myself, that we don't seem to think or know now?

So What Now?

It might surprise you that my reaction to all this is, "So?" There's only one obvious problem here, and there's a simple (I didn't say easy) solution: a lot of us collectively forgot to wear the "suit," and what there is to do is put it back on. For (probably) the last time in this book: When adults meet children's needs for affirmation, information, clarity about values, limit-setting, and anticipatory guidance, they thrive. And when we don't, they don't.

The excellent news is that the Internet itself is full of solutions. There are dozens of terrific resources (see the family resources list) with kid-tested suggestions for affirming and supporting children's need and desire to learn and play online, while making those experiences safe and constructive. If your children are quite young, you've got the advantage. You can without question establish your power and authority over *all* electronic devices in your home and the rules that govern them (I remember when children of any age were required to ask permission before turning on the TV) and create a plan going forward for increasing your kids' freedom and options as they earn them. Go ahead: stamp each and every device with the mantra "Independence is earned."

You'll have to hang tough because of the pressure that begin as early as kindergarten, if not before. The five-year-old daughter of a mom I know was invited to a birthday party. When the mom learned that pictures of the party and the children attending were going to be posted on the family's networking page, she simply declined the invite. She had just read about facial recognition software that networking sites use, and didn't want her daughter exposed, and also wanted to insulate her from the idea of social networking as kids' play. Here's where networking among parents even of young kids can really pay off. It's simply too easy to get carried off by every enticing new wave of possibilities that technology continually creates; parents can help one another keep their common sense—and their primary focus on children and their needs—intact.

If your kids are older, say fourth to eighth grade, they may be used to more leeway. If you want to reconsider and rein in the use of electronic devices, well, who says parents can't change their mind about the best way to parent? (If you're shaking your head and thinking your kids won't go along, remind yourself who paid for and still owns all of those devices in the first place; if you remain firm, they'll *have* to go along if they want access at all.) It's a very good idea—I personally would go so far as to say it's imperative—to move the computer to a public space if it's not already there, and to give your children a set number of recreational "screen time" hours per week for *all* screens in your home—including cell phones, and even devices they may have bought with their own money—to budget as they please.

Think, too, about establishing screen-free days for the entire family (if that idea personally makes you break a sweat, all the more reason to consider it), and talk to your kids frequently about the values and rules you expect them to bring to all of their online experiences, including at other families' homes. Here are two basic rules of thumb for kids of all ages: (1) The same rules that apply to treatment of others in person apply, always, to any form of Internet communication, too. (2) Don't write or post any words or images online you wouldn't want your grandmother to read or see, because she might. Let them know that you'll need access to any passwords they create, and that you'll be looking periodically at their online settings, Internet history, and, if they're allowed to have one, the contents of their social networking page.

You'll need to tell them your reasons for all the rules, old and new, and also what behaviors you'll look for in deciding when to give them more freedom. (This all sounds very familiar, right?) Be sure to make the point that the policy will continue when they start high school; that independence will always be earned; and that you consider the use of technology for recreational purposes a privilege, not an entitlement.

For high school kids, making change can get dicey. If they've had few restrictions so far, they may feel entitled to use technology however they see fit, since that has been the case in the past and why should it change, especially now that they're older? Unless they've broken other rules or they've been involved on the Internet in an unsafe or abusive way that warrants taking away their privileges, it's easy to end up in an unwinnable power struggle if you suddenly try to take too much control. Regardless, you can always be very direct with your teens about your *expectations* regarding their use of technology, even if you lack the means to enforce specific rules. Stating our clear expectations is one of the most important ways we *maintain influence* on teenagers' decisions, even as kids get older and we inevitably lose some of our power.

Here's the other leverage you always have: Chances are, if teenagers are spending too much time online, texting, or with other activities or forms of technology, their homework, grades, applications, jobs, sports commitments, relationships, sleep, exercise, time spent with family, or other important activities or responsibilities are getting short shrift. You still have *plenty* of say over anything—including technology—that directly affects their physical, social, or emotional health. Very often, high school kids who are in over their heads are relieved when adults step in to help them get their life back into better control by changing habits they've not been able to change on their own.[13]

All families should take a page out of what most schools and businesses do. When your kids are as young as possible—and with their input—develop a written Family Acceptable Use Policy (AUP), with some parts applicable to everyone in the family, including the adults.[14] The policy, signed by everyone, should cover every technological device in your home, from TVs to tablets, with specific rules about what they may be used for and not, and when. Make it a "living" document that you and your kids alter (and re-sign) through ongoing negotiations. It won't put you in the driver's seat, where you don't really want to be anyway, but it surely will enable you to keep one hand—as firmly or lightly as need be—on the wheel. Check out the family resource list in the back of this book for excellent guidance and resources on creating an AUP that will suit your particular family's needs.

One last thought: I'm personally not a fan of "parental controls," because I think it's a misnomer and a wrongheaded idea. Relying on technology to police itself misses the point, since it enables parents to actually give away responsibility *and* control. Better, I think, is a hands-on approach, such as an AUP, because it enables us to monitor our kids and teaches them gradually how to monitor themselves. Also, keep in mind that the same filters also screen out really helpful information from reliable sites about topics such as sexuality that we may indeed want them to learn how to access. And of course, most of our computer-savvy teens and preteens can figure out, or find out at will, how to get around the controls. Without previous, incremental guidance on managing the Internet's "unbridled freedom," they'll be left to fend on their own.

Talking About Pornography

I rarely say things this prescriptively, but here goes: *all* parents need to talk to their children about pornography. If your children or teens have access to the Internet, it's practically inevitable they'll stumble onto sexually explicit material, view it with a friend, or follow their curiosity and deliberately seek it out. At the very least, sooner or later they will hear about it from peers.

Here's where laying the groundwork will really serve you well in getting there first. (I would suggest fourth or fifth grade.) If your children know how the sexual system of the body works—that it's a part of their nervous system that produces sexual pleasure and that it's responsive to thoughts, touch, sight, and other senses, too—it will seem logical if you explain that some people like to look at "sexy" images or videos of people "sexing" (see how nicely that word works) because it gives their bodies pleasure. Still pictures or video that arouses those feelings is called pornography or "porn." There are thousands and thousands of companies that make pornography and sell it to grown-ups on the Internet, and to get their attention, they even know how to make it "pop up" suddenly on a computer. "If you ever come across pornography," you can say, "come and tell me, because it's intended for grown-ups, not children."

The message I would give younger children, as part of a larger conversation about rules for the Internet, is something like this: "Sometimes children see pictures or videos on a computer that really surprise or shock them. They might even see naked people who are kissing or touching other naked people. Come and talk to me right away if that ever happens." Not exactly the kind of anticipatory guidance we would like to have to give, but we're obliged to raise children in the world as it is.

As for talking to teens, here's a revealing anecdote: A parent once called me after discovering by accident that her teenage son had been viewing pornography online. "That's okay, right?" she wanted to know. "He's naturally curious and sooner or later he needs to know about sex, so why not?" What she hadn't considered, and didn't think to explain to her son, is there's more to pornography than "sex." The important issue, particularly for young people, is *how the sex is commonly portrayed.*

First of all, all young people need to understand that pornography is essentially fake. It's a scripted performance, in no way natural or a reflection of real life. In real life, a sexual experience is for and about the two people involved—in fact, isn't that the point? Pornography, on the other hand, is for and about the camera, the competition, and the paying customer; the more outrageous the advertised and depicted behaviors, the better the prospects for sales. Teens who are uninformed may think what they see is the norm and may pressure themselves, their peers, or their sexual partners to perform in these ways, too.

What's more, the actors' bodies in pornographic images are hardly average or typical, many altered or distorted by plastic surgery or hormones. (Requests for female genital cosmetic surgery, including labiaplasty and clitoral unhooding, are on the increase, as more and more women, and even teenage girls, now express dissatisfaction with the appearance of their vulvas.[15] A significant contributing factor is thought to be unrealistic standards of "perfection" created for men and women by these pornographic images, compounded by widespread ignorance about the normal variation in size and shape of these parts. Sadly, insecurity about the appearance of perfectly normal genitals is no longer the exclusive domain of boys and men.) The interaction between the characters is impersonal *by definition*—after all, it is just a job—and rarely equal in terms of power and control. Though not all pornography is deliberately demeaning, most often women's bodies are shown in degrading and humiliating positions, with the implication that women exist to service and provide pleasure for men, and that men enjoy using them for selfish gain. Even more troubling is the abundance of rape imagery in pornography that is readily accessible. Perhaps worse than the implied violence is the total absence of empathy, remorse, or accountability, thereby implicitly validating a dehumanizing and dangerous connection between cruelty and sex.

Especially for highly curious, impressionable teenagers, typically with little or no life experience to form a reasonable basis for comparison, the very real concern is that exposure to pornography will promote a distorted set of perceptions and expectations—unless, of course, we adults get there first with a serious reality check. The fact that pornography is so widely available offers *all* parents a logical opening to bring up the subject with *all* teens, not just with those we know have *already* been exposed. (In fact, if you've discovered pornography on your child's computer, you needn't even bring that up.) Remember, the issue isn't sex, but children's need for anticipatory guidance *about* sex; these conversations give all parents the opportunity to reinforce—by way of comparison—what *we* want our kids to understand about the nature and meaning of sex.

When I ask teens to tell me why they think their parents don't want them to look at pornography, they most often say, "Because adults don't want us to know about sex." What an opening to explain that there's a whole lot more to pornography than sex, and a whole lot more to sex than pornography.

Reprise: The Forest and the Tree

The call from the woman about her son and pornography was typical of many I receive. When sex enters the picture, as we've said, Americans have trouble seeing beyond the sexual content to the *context* in which it occurs.

A case in point is "freaking" or "grinding," the dancing kids do that involves rubbing genitals to genitals, or genitals to rears, and sometimes both, with one person wedged between two others he or she may not even know. Some people describe it as simulated sex. (I say, if kids are rubbing their genitals together, and feeling sexually aroused, there's nothing "simulated" about it.) I remember the first call I received about grinding in the mid-1990s from a teacher who'd just seen it at a twelfth-grade dance. She said, "What gives, and why doesn't anyone seem to care about this but me?"

The truth is, adults did care but didn't know what to do. They knew it was sexual, but kids had their clothes on and weren't really "having sex." They knew they were uncomfortable but couldn't explain to themselves exactly why. They couldn't imagine talking to kids about it, or how. They looked around at other adults, who seemed to be okay with it. So, most just stood on the sidelines, pretending it was okay with them, too. And the next year eleventh graders were doing it, too. And so on.

The adults couldn't get to the issue at stake because it was about values and context, not "sex"; explicit sexuality—and the anxiety it provoked—was the tree that was blocking their view. If we want kids to associate sexual experiences with particular values—such as privacy, intimacy, and respect for boundaries, time, and place—we need to take a stand on their behalf. First we have to be able to see beyond the "sex" to the context beyond; then we can explain what our objections are really about and set limits accordingly.

One summer I met a twenty-year-old college student who was a DJ on the side. He'd been shocked to spot *fifth graders* grinding at a graduation party in a public elementary school the previous spring. He was even more surprised that the parents and teachers did nothing about it. "What did you do?" I asked. "I turned off the music and told them to stop, and they did." Sometimes it's that simple.

"Sexting"

If you are ever looking for a great topic to nurture about and around, "sexting" would be it.[16] Let's start with "the media." By distilling this issue down to a catchy (and sexy) seven-letter buzzword, the media have managed, again, to reduce a hugely complex phenomenon to its least common denominator: "reckless teenagers sending nude/sexy pictures and having their lives ruined and even going to jail." As Andrew Harris, a professor of criminology at the University of Massachusetts, put it, "We're talking [here] about a lot of different behaviors and a lot of different motivations": flirting, attention-seeking, consensual exchanges between adults, teenagers "horsing" around, pressure from a boyfriend or girlfriend, revenge, malicious distribution, and even extortion."[17] (A boy in Wisconsin in 2009 pretended to be a girl and solicited nude pictures of other boys so he could blackmail them.) If ever a subject deserved *not* to be reduced to a sound bite, this would be it.

There are countless "ways in" for parents of teens of all ages about topics this complex; that's the good news about media hype, if we take the time to "unpack" it (and don't let it scare us into overreacting). By simply drawing upon current news stories[18] and asking good questions, we can help ensure that our kids won't think in sound bites, even if that's all they hear elsewhere. And if we're conscious and conscientious about it, in the process of asking we can make sure to touch base with all five needs/roles in one conversation. For example, affirmation: "There are healthier and safer ways to get someone's attention. What are some reasons, do you think, someone might choose this one?" Information: "As they say, the Internet 'never forgets.' What could be some consequences, immediate and in the future, of sending or posting this kind of stuff?" Clarity about values: "More often than not, it's girls who are sending nude photos and boys requesting them. Does that seem like a double standard to you? Who has more to gain or lose, do you think?" Limits: "Yes, by law in some states, this really is considered child pornography. I'm curious to know what you think about that." Anticipatory guidance: "In what kinds of situations might it be hard to say no to something like this, even if you knew it would be stupid or wrong?" Wondering out loud with your daughter or son about all of these dynamics, with no purpose other than to stimulate good thinking and conversation, makes them stronger and wiser. Have a crack at it!

Turning Our Children over to Themselves

When he was approaching his senior year, I took my younger son on a college visit to Chicago. It was a glorious early summer day, and we walked and walked, soaking up the sunshine and beauty of the city. (I didn't have the heart to tell him what it would look and feel like in the dead of winter.) We talked a lot about the coming changes in his life, and at some point it occurred to him to ask, "Mom, is there anything else you forgot to tell me about life that I really need to know?"

Reminiscing about that moment recently, the two of us shared a huge laugh. If only growing up, and parenting, was that simple! No matter how much we would like to continue to pave their way, there are things about life our children will begin to learn only when it's fully *their* life to live, and when we are truly on the sidelines. What we teach them, before they and we let go, will go only that far. But if we're fully aware and conscious about nurturing them in all the ways they need and want, we can feel ever more confident and proud about turning them over to themselves.

And oh, by the way, that applies to sexuality, too.

9

Practice Makes Proficient:
Let's Go Fishing

To complete a differential diagnosis in a confusing or complicated case, doctors take a history, run a battery of tests, and examine the patient's body. In the end, they may still end up having to take a highly educated best guess from among several possibilities. Parents are lucky: in sorting through what a child needs in *any* situation, there are only five possibilities, and they're always the same.

Here are some final scenarios to help you practice discerning which one or more needs—affirmation, information, clarity about values, limit-setting, and/or anticipatory guidance—is present in any given situation. (Hint: whenever you're in doubt, start with affirmation.) Each of them is a real-life example. Some of them will likely stir personal reactions, so identify and think or write about those before moving on to the next one, since it's always best in those situations to start by trying to separate your needs from your child's. Then jot down the needs you identify, and possible responses.

Is That . . . a Vibrator?

You ask your fifteen-year-old daughter where she put the sweater she borrowed from you. She tells you to check the middle drawer of her dresser. In the drawer, right under the sweater, you spot a vibrator.

1. Your immediate thoughts and feelings:
2. What does your child want in the situation? What is your child thinking or feeling?
3. What does your child need from you in the situation? What are your roles?
4. What you would say and/or do:

Who Owns the Car Radio?

Your eight- and eleven-going-on-twelve-year-old sons are in the car on an hourlong trip. Your older son turns on the radio to his favorite radio station and suddenly you hear song lyrics laced with sexual references and sexist language. You say, "Please change the channel," and he says, "Dad, every kid I know listens to this channel, and in their cars, too, with their parents driving them. I've been there, so I'm not making this up."

1. Your immediate thoughts and feelings:
2. What does your child want in the situation? What is your child thinking or feeling?
3. What does your child need from you in the situation? What are your roles?
4. What you would say and/or do:

Where Did You Learn to Move Like That?

Your six-year-old daughter is posing, strutting, and moving her hips in ways that are very "sexy." She clearly enjoys the positive attention she receives from people who think it's "cute."

1. Your immediate thoughts and feelings:
2. What does your child want in the situation? What is your child thinking or feeling?
3. What does your child need from you in the situation? What are your roles?
4. What you would say and/or do:

Ouch, That Hurts!

You have two daughters, an infant and a three-year-old. Sometimes when you sit down to nurse the baby, the three-year-old comes over and pinches your breast.

1. Your immediate thoughts and feelings:
2. What does your child want in the situation? What is your child thinking or feeling?
3. What does your child need from you in the situation? What are your roles?
4. What you would say and/or do?

Self-Pleasuring . . . in Church?

For the second week in a row, your four-year-old son starts rubbing his penis halfway into the pastor's sermon. The last time it went on for ten minutes.

1. Your immediate thoughts and feelings:
2. What does your child want in the situation? What is your child thinking or feeling?
3. What does your child need from you in the situation? What are your roles?
4. What you would say and/or do:

How Old Were You
When You First Had Sex?

Your fourteen-year-old asks how old you were for your "first time."

1. Your immediate thoughts and feelings:
2. What does your child want in the situation? What is your child thinking or feeling?
3. What does your child need from you in the situation? What are your roles?
4. What you would say and/or do:

Under My Roof?

Your sixteen-year-old bisexual daughter has a girlfriend. Her girlfriend is planning to sleep overnight.

1. Your immediate thoughts and feelings:
2. What does your child want in the situation? What is your child thinking or feeling?
3. What does your child need from you in the situation? What are your roles?
4. What you would say and/or do:

Under My Roof? (Redux)

Your sophomore son comes home from college, bringing his new girlfriend with him. You know they spend nights together at school. When they come in, they both take their suitcases to his room. (Play it out two ways: one where there are other siblings in your home, and one where there aren't.)

1. Your immediate thoughts and feelings:
2. What does your child want in the situation? What is your child thinking or feeling?

3. What does your child need from you in the situation? What are your roles?
4. What you would say and/or do:

"Losing" Your Virginity

You hear your fifteen-going-on-sixteen-year-old daughter crying in her room. You ask to come in and she finally tells you what's wrong. Her boyfriend just broke up with her. She starts really sobbing when she tells you, "And I lost my virginity with him, too!"

1. Your immediate thoughts and feelings:
2. What does your child want in the situation? What is your child thinking or feeling?
3. What does your child need from you in the situation? What are your roles?
4. What you would say and/or do:

Here are some possible responses, and things to think about, drawing on principles in this book. They're meant only as teasers to give you, perhaps, an alternative point of view, or validation that you know how to consciously wear the "suit." Only you know your personal values, your life circumstances, and your kids, and only you can determine what's best. That's the point, remember, of your getting there first.

Is That . . . a Vibrator?

Finding a vibrator in your teenage daughter's drawer could certainly put you to the test as few things can. You might think, intellectually, *Well, yes, I believe in girls' right to know and enjoy their bodies, and to take responsibility for their own sexual pleasure.* Yet, this kind of discovery might push every single one of your buttons about your daughter's sexuality—and possibly your own—giving you much to contemplate. Let it be an opportunity to clarify your own values and feelings. Parenting asks that of us all the time about all kinds of subjects. It would also be good to be especially aware of any projections that surface on your part about what else your daughter might be doing sexually that you don't know about, and also to do a reality check on whatever anxiety you may be experiencing.

As for your daughter, I think I would go with *affirmation* in this case, by respecting her privacy. I would wonder, though, if she'll realize that you might have seen what was in the drawer, so I would be especially attentive the next few days, and if she looks as though there's something on her mind, I would probably reflect that back to her ("You seem like there's something on your mind. Anything you want to talk about?") and give her an opening to bring it up. I would think carefully in advance, though, about what you want to say if she asks your opinion. If not, and if you're still feeling as if she's worried about your reaction to what you may have seen, simply look for special opportunities to validate her and show her your love and acceptance. You might also think about bringing up a related issue—there are media and even news references all the time to the topic of sexual pleasure—and speak about it in an even, positive tone.

Who Owns the Car Radio?

What an easy question: *you do,* of course, and can do with it as you please. You've got a couple of good choices, though I do have a preference. You can decide to set a limit—"No, we're going to find something else"—though I would take it a couple of steps further. I would want to explain why I feel the way I do, and name the values I hold that the lyrics contradict. By having them on in my car, I would explain, I would feel I was giving a stamp of approval to ideas I abhor. I would also challenge his normative beliefs about what "all kids" and "all parents" do. Option B is the one I would prefer, especially now that I know this kind of music is part of his social life. I would say, "Here's the ticket. The reception on this channel is going to run out in about twenty minutes. We'll listen until it goes, and then we'll talk together for the rest of the trip about the words in the lyrics, what they mean, and why many people, including me, find them upsetting. Why don't you write down some of the words while we're listening." As for the younger sibling in the back, I would include him from time to time to hear his opinions, too.

Where Did You Learn to Move Like That?

To me, this one's a straightforward case of limit-setting. You can say firmly (no need for conversation here, just clear limit-setting), "That's the way some women might walk. Since you're a child, not a grown-up, show me how little children walk."

Ouch, That Hurts!

This seems like another situation requiring a straightforward statement, such as "Don't pinch my breast. That really hurts!" For some parents, cases like this one are not so clear-cut. The woman who shared this scenario with me about her daughter Jackie was really stuck about what to do, because she'd misread the need. She'd confused Jackie's need for *limit-setting* with her need for *affirmation*. "I really want her to think of breasts as positive," she told me. "If I tell her to stop, won't she think I'm saying they're bad?" (Would her worry be the same if Jackie had pinched her arm?) Affirming sexuality doesn't mean saying yes to everything, especially when there's such an obvious cost. It was time to set a limit, and worry about affirming "positive breast image" at another time in another way.

Jackie does seem to need affirmation, but in a different way. Very likely she's letting Mom know how jealous and angry she feels about the new baby. After all, a rival for Mom's all-important attention had just suddenly appeared. Mom's breasts are a logical target for her feelings, since whenever the baby is nursing, Jackie must feel like the odd girl out. Some special alone time with Jackie each day would likely curb her aggression, especially if Mom was clear it must stop.

Sometimes a cigar is just a cigar, and a breast is just, well, convenient.

Self-Pleasuring . . . in Church?

Most adults today know it's normal for young children to soothe themselves by stroking their genitals whenever they feel anxious or sleepy or bored. But do they have to do it in church? Well, yes. They don't yet comprehend concepts such as privacy, or the appropriateness of proper time and place. So, it's not as though you can say on the way to the service, "You know, touching your genitals is a private behavior, so please, can you get it all in now?" Best to ignore it, and teach those lessons when the child is ready, usually sometime between five and six. If you won't last that long—or even the next ten seconds—just get up with your child and go for a walk.

How Old Were You When You First Had Sex?

Don't let personal questions about sex make you squirm. It's a perfect nurturing opportunity, and an example of how well you can start out with one need (in this case, seemingly, for information) and expand the conversation to touch on all five. (And by the way, you don't even have to answer the question.)

Parents are often conflicted about whether they should be totally honest with their kids about their personal decisions and experiences. My one rule of thumb is there should always be a point to your openness: What did you learn from the experience, and how would it help your child if you shared it? When it comes to sexuality, though, I think you have a right to take a pass whenever you want. After all, one of the important messages kids today need to hear from their parents is that sexual experiences are intended to be personal and private, and that they also involve another person's privacy. Saying, "I'm not comfortable talking about that because it's too private," is as much of an honest and open response as spilling all the details. And it's not a cop-out either, if it's the simple truth.

But you don't have to leave it at that. Probably your child isn't interested in your sex life at all, but *how you made decisions* about it. You can always add, "Let's play out the question. How would you feel if I said fourteen, sixteen, twenty-one, or twenty-four? What do you think is a good age, and how do you know?" In the process, you can provide or reinforce good information (sex isn't only intercourse; there are all kinds of "firsts," and they are really important to think about, too); clarify values (ask your child what would be important to her or him in a sexual relationship, including each important "first"); state limits (here's what I think are the minimum ages, and why); and anticipatory guidance (sexual experiences can be positive or negative at any age; here are the things to keep in mind).

Under My Roof? (Part 1)

No matter your child's sexual orientation, this is an enlightening example; as a brain-teaser, it's a winner. The last time I asked a group of parents to think through the scenario together, they became immersed in more questions and more confusion than when they set out: Well, suppose she wanted to bring home a boyfriend; how would that change things? Nobody can get pregnant in this situation. Does that change how it should be viewed? Girls sleep in the same room, even in the same bed, and get undressed in front of each other all the time. How is that different in this situation and in what ways does it matter? Would we insist that our daughters be as careful in their sexual choices if they were lesbians? How about our gay sons?

In the end, the group decided to find a core principle and stick with it all the way through: Spending the night together as a romantic couple is a privilege reserved for adults. Alone time together can happen at other times, as a form of independence that young people earn. What do you think?

Under My Roof? (Part 2)

When older children come home to visit, they often bring an odd mixture of joy and conflict for parents. We're so glad to see them, *and* we'll probably need to renegotiate some rules. In this particular example, whenever possible, it's good to have these conversations in advance, to avoid an unnecessary or awkward confrontation.

Once again, I see really clear options, and all of them revolve around *your* needs and values, not your son's. (Your son and his girlfriend might *want* to sleep in the same room, but they don't *need* to, so you're off the hook.) For some parents, having the two of them sleep in the same bedroom may seem perfectly fine and natural. For others, it could be a source of great discomfort, even an affront to deeply held beliefs. It's your home! There could be a downside, however, you might want to consider: in option B, your son might not be so eager to come home.

For other parents the issue isn't sex, but integrity. If you've made it clear all along that sleeping in the same room is a privilege for grown-ups, and if your son has been living at least somewhat independently on his own, allowing the two to stay together might seem perfectly consistent. What's more, if you know they spend nights together at school, if might seem like dishonesty or pretense not to allow it in your home.

"Losing" Your Virginity

First, some background: Kids today still regard "virginity" as a defining concept in their lives, even though many of today's attitudes toward virginity date back thousands of years. The concept of virginity has deep religious and spiritual meaning for many people, still, because they consider premarital chastity a sacred value. Moreover, before people knew how to effectively practice birth control, virginity was emphasized also as a kind of insurance policy against premarital pregnancy; people make that same argument today, in regard both to pregnancy *and* STI/HIV prevention.

There's a third historical piece that is generally less well known and understood. It has to do with the historical status of girls and women as "property." Throughout much of history, and tragically, in many places in the world even today, a young woman's only real worth to her community was her ability to produce male heirs who could later inherit their father's property and wealth. Her virginity upon marriage was considered absolutely essential, since it was vitally important for her to remain totally faithful to her husband to ensure that the babies she produced were *his* babies. Hence the term "loss of virginity." In many cultures, if an unmarried female was even suspected of not being a virgin, she stood to lose virtually everything, including her worth as a human being, and maybe even her life, because she would no longer be considered marriageable.

This last bit of history is important for parents to understand because it will help them and their children think through the importance and meaning of virginity in their own lives. First of all, we live in an age and a place where women and men are officially equal from a legal perspective, and girls and women are considered worthy human beings in countless ways. I like to challenge my students to think deeply about the phrase "loss of virginity" (which they apply to both girls and boys), the kinds of attitudes it reflects, and their relevance in the world in which they live. Why not frame sexual experiences in terms of what people stand to gain, for example, not what they stand to lose? Words are powerful, and they help shape the way people make decisions, think about their options, and take responsibility for possible gains *and* losses.

Back to the scenario: Upon hearing what your daughter has said, you may indeed need time to process the information she has just given you. Best to hold that in check, if you can. Go-to people have to be prepared for whatever their children may bring.

In the moment, what she needs most of all is affirmation, best provided by your listening deeply and without judgment to her thoughts and feelings. What a precious gift she has just given you—her trust in you to do precisely that. There will be time later for you to give her the information, clarity about values, limits, and guidance she'll need to make healthy—or healthier, if that's the case—decisions.

And Finally, a Post-Test

Here are eight additional scenarios to try out on your own. For each one, see if you can find a way to touch on all five needs in one conversation: affirmation, information, clarity about values, limit-setting, and anticipatory guidance.

Crazy for Cheerleaders

At a promotional event sponsored by your local professional football team, one of the cheerleaders gave your seven-year-old son cards with individual pictures of her and other cheerleaders dressed in the revealing costumes they wear at games. He's fascinated by the images and now constantly talks about "boobies." It's getting almost to the point of obsession.

1. Your immediate thoughts and feelings:
2. What does your child want in the situation? What is your child thinking or feeling?
3. What does your child need from you in the situation? What are your roles?
4. What you would say and/or do:

I Don't Want to Do It Anymore (Part 1)

You're the father of a seventeen-year-old boy. He says to you, "Dad, you said I could talk to you about anything, right? I'm feeling really bad about myself. Some of my friends at school have been playing up to younger girls and getting them to give them blow jobs. The girls think we really like them. I've done it, too, a couple of times. I know it's not right. How do I get myself out of this?"

1. Your immediate thoughts and feelings:
2. What does your child want in the situation? What is your child thinking or feeling?
3. What does your child need from you in the situation? What are your roles?
4. What you would say and/or do:

I Don't Want to Do It Anymore (Part 2)

You're the father of a six-year-old. He comes to tell you that he's feeling bad about something. A friend, slightly older and generally a more aggressive child, has wanted him to rub his penis several times. He hasn't done it but did let the other boy rub his. He knows this is wrong. He is tearing up.

1. Your immediate thoughts and feelings:
2. What does your child want in the situation? What is your child thinking or feeling?
3. What does your child need from you in the situation? What are your roles?
4. What you would say and/or do:

"That's So Gay"

Kids in your car pool constantly say, "That's so gay," when they mean that something is "stupid" or "weird," or "he's so gay," when they mean another child is a "loser." Once you asked them to stop, and one of the kids said, "Oh, we don't mean gay as in a gay *person*. We don't have anything against gay people. It's just the way we talk. It doesn't mean anything." Your child does not join in but seems to take it all in.

1. Your immediate thoughts and feelings:
2. What does your child want in the situation? What is your child thinking or feeling?
3. What does your child need from you in the situation? What are your roles?
4. What you would say and/or do:

Does Sex Hurt?

Your thirteen-year-old asks you, "Does sex hurt?"

1. Your immediate thoughts and feelings:
2. What does your child want in the situation? What is your child thinking or feeling?
3. What does your child need from you in the situation? What are your roles?
4. What you would say and/or do:

OOOPS

Your four-year-old wanders into your room late at night and comes across you and your partner/spouse engaging in very obvious sexual activity.

1. Your immediate thoughts and feelings:
2. What does your child want in the situation? What is your child thinking or feeling?
3. What does your child need from you in the situation? What are your roles?
4. What you would say and/or do:

OOOPS (Redux)

Your seven-year-old wanders into your room late at night and comes across you and your partner/spouse engaging in very obvious sexual activity.

1. Your immediate thoughts and feelings:
2. What does your child want in the situation? What is your child thinking or feeling?
3. What does your child need from in the situation? What are your roles?
4. What you would say and/or do: (right after your bug zapper goes off and you say, "What do you mean by 'sex'?"):

What's the Right Age for Sex?

Your twelve-year-old asks you this question, just after you've expressed your disapproval of a scenario involving teenagers and sex on a TV show you're both watching.

1. Your immediate thoughts and feelings:
2. What does your child want in the situation? What is your child thinking or feeling?
3. What does your child need from you in the situation? What are your roles?
4. What you would say and/or do (right after your bug zapper goes off and you ask what she means by "sex"):

Time Alone with Boyfriend

Your sixteen-year-old daughter has a steady boyfriend. She's a really responsible high school student. So is he. You know and like his parents. So far, the two of them have never been alone in either of your homes for any length of time. She says, "Can Ronald come over to study with me tomorrow for the math test on Friday?" You say, "Sorry, but no. You know the rules." She says, because of how you've taught her to think, "How can I show you that I've earned this privilege?"

1. Your immediate thoughts and feelings:
2. What does your child want in the situation? What is your child thinking or feeling?
3. What does your child need from you in the situation? What are your roles?
4. What you would say and/or do:

Epilogue

There you have it. My hope is that you come away from *Talk to Me First* feeling more self-assured, adept, and most of all excited about embracing the role of sexuality educator-in-chief in your kids' lives. I also hope that you will find much joy and fulfillment in the conversations to come.

I ask that if you can, please take steps to give away what you know. In today's world, it will take whole communities of savvy, motivated, and involved parents (and teachers) to nurture a next generation of sexually healthy children, adolescents, and adults. So, talk to and support one another in "wearing the suit"; make hard phone calls; help ensure that adults aren't afraid of the wrong things, such as information from caring adults; encourage a common language around "values" and a common stance around age-appropriate limits and boundaries; start a book club or help your school initiate grade-level parents' meetings; have one another's backs when children's safety and well-being are at stake; explain the importance of "educating for yes," not "no" or "not yet"; and/or advocate for truly comprehensive sexuality education at your children's schools, and form school/family partnerships to strengthen our overlapping yet unique roles.

Let's, all of us, help bring American culture into the twenty-first century around meeting children's and adolescents' real and pressing needs in regard to their healthy sexual development. As I wrote in Chapter 1, we really don't have another decade to waste.

Acknowledgments

Writing a book is intensely personal. It's all about you and your keyboard for hours on end, days and weeks at a time. (Thank goodness for my dog, who faithfully kept me company.) It's also about putting yourself—and only yourself—on the line, personally and professionally. At times it can be lonely and intimidating. But for almost everyone who enjoys putting words to a page and who feels blessed by the opportunity to toss her ideas and experiences into the public arena, every minute is worth it.

What readers don't get to see or know are all the people in your life who helped make you who you are, and who supported you every step of the way from the first day you sat down to write.

My first and most heartfelt acknowledgment is to my husband, David, who has been my best friend and biggest cheerleader through more than forty years of marriage. He has spent almost as many hours alone during this project as I, and taken on my half of the responsibilities of running our household to boot, without an ounce of resentment (I think) and with good humor. What would I do without you?

Second, I want to thank my editor at Perseus Books Group, Renee Sedliar, for believing in this project from the moment I pitched it, and for waving her magical wand over my drafts with such brilliance, precision, and sensitivity. To Lissa Warren, my longtime publicist at Perseus, what a joy and privilege it has been to know and work with you. Many thanks, too, to Cisca Schreefel, project editor for *Talk to Me First*, for her graciousness and skillful guidance. My deep gratitude goes as well to Jim Dale and Kathy Shapiro for setting me on the right path by helping me frame my original book proposal.

The Park School of Baltimore, where I have worked since 1975, is truly my home away from home. To everyone I've worked with at Park—students, teachers, administrators, staff, and parents—there are no words to express how important you are to me. I would especially like to say thanks to my colleagues on the Health Team and Park Connects Team—Dave Tracey, Zella Adams, Krista Dhruv, Jan Brant, Ellen Small, and Patti Flowers-Coulson. All of you have taught me enough about parenting and kids to fill volumes. Many thanks, too, to Christopher Mergen for his amazing assistance with portions of the manuscript, and to Marla Hollandsworth and Rich Espey for their very sensitive and sensible guidance as well. Over the years, Hillary Jacobs, former director of communications, has been a source of tremendous support, for which I will always be grateful. And to Bev Kempler, who asks me every day how things are going and really wants to know, thanks for always being there.

Many people reviewed portions of the manuscript and offered invaluable input: Peggy Brick, Joan Garrity, Dr. Jennifer Bryan, Dr. Chris Kraft, Deborah Mitnick, Dave Tracey, Zella Adams, Adam Roffman, Shira Wallach, and Julie Levison. Thanks to Krista Dhruv and Patti Flowers-Coulson for your wizardry with online research. A huge shout-out goes to my son Josh, who read and reviewed each and every chapter, and to my son Adam, who has been solving my computer problems ever since he was four.

Notes

Chapter 1

1. Strickland, A. "Adult-Inspired Lingerie Marketed for Young Girls." CNN.com, www .cnn.com/2011/LIVING/08/18/young.girls.lingerie/index.html?iref=allsearch; Malken, S. "Not So Pretty in Pink: Marketing Toxic Makeup to Young Girls." January 15, 2009, http://archive.truthout.org/011409wa?.

Chapter 2

1. Irvine, M. "10 Is the New 15 as Kids Grow Up Faster." *USA Today*, November 26, 2006.

2. Pollet, A., and P. Hurwitz. "Strip Till You Drop: Teen Girls Are the Target Market for a New Wave of Stripper Inspired Merchandise." *The Nation*, January 12/19, 2005, pages 20–25; Orenstein, P. "The Empowerment Mystique: What's Being Sold in Ads Promoting Female Pride?" *New York Times Magazine*, September 26, 2010, page 11.

3. Goldstein, L. "Church Report Cites Social Tumult in Priest Scandals." *New York Times*, May 17, 2011.

4. Straus, M., and E. McCollum. "Resisting Madison Avenue's Manipulations." *Networker*, March/April 2000, pages 55–56.

5. Kantrowitz, B., and P. Wingert. "The Truth About Tweens." *Newsweek*, October 18, 1999, pages 61–69, 72.

6. Chmielewski, D. "How Disney Tapped into the Tween Market." *Los Angeles Times*, July 1, 2009, www.heraldextra.com/entertainment/arts-and-theatre/kids-and-teens/article_9350 4267-9322-58b4-a130-51df0bf3c7e3.html.

7. Hoffman, J. "Masculinity in a Spray Can." *New York Times*, January 31, 2010, www.ny times.com/2010/01/31/fashion/31smell.html?pagewanted=all.

8. Ruskin, G. "Why They Whine: How Corporations Prey on Our Children." *Mothering Magazine*, November/December 1999; Beder, S. "Marketing to Children" in *A Community View, Caring for Children in the Media Age*, papers from a national conference, edited by John Squires and Tracy Newlands, New College Institute for Values Research, Sydney, 1998, pages 101–111; http://herinst.org/sbeder/children/children.html; Zoll, M. "Psychologists Challenge Ethics of Marketing to Children." American News Service, April 5, 2000, www.berkshire publishing.com/ans/HTMView.asp?parItem=S031000377A; Norris, M. "Advertisers Target Adult Products to Children." *World News Tonight*, ABC News, May 10, 2002; American Psychology Association. "Driving Teen Egos—and Buying—Through 'Branding.'" *Monitor on Psychology* 35, no. 6 (June 2004): 60; www.apa.org/monitor/jun04/driving.aspx.

9. Tyre, P., J. Scelfo, and B. Kantrowitz. "The Power of No." *Newsweek*, September 13, 2004, pages 42–50; Kindlon, D. *Too Much of a Good Thing: Raising Children of Character in an Indulgent Age.* New York: Hyperion, 2001.

Chapter 3

1. Gordon, T. *PET: Parent Effectiveness Training.* New York: Peter H. Wyden, 1970.

Chapter 4

1. Fausto-Sterling, A. *Sexing the Body: Gender Politics and the Construction of Sexuality.* New York: Basic Books, 2000.

2. Roffman, D. M. *Sex and Sensibility: The Thinking Parent's Guide to Talking Sense About Sex.* Boston: Da Capo Press, 2001.

Chapter 5

1. Bernstein, A. *Flight of the Stork: What Children Think (and When) About Sex and Family Building.* Indianapolis: Perspective Press, 1994; Roffman, D. M. *But How'd I Get in There in the First Place?: Talking to Your Young Child About Sex.* Boston: Da Capo Press, 2002; National Guidelines Task Force. *Guidelines for Comprehensive Sexuality Education,* kindergarten to twelfth grade. New York: Sexuality Information and Education Council of the United States (SIECUS), 1996; Johnson, T. C. *Understanding Your Child's Sexual Behavior: What's Natural and Healthy.* Oakland, CA: New Harbinger Publications, 1999.

Chapter 6

1. Fletcher, J. *Situational Ethics: The New Morality.* Louisville, KY: Westminster John Knox Press, 1966.

2. Brooks, D. "If It Feels Right . . ." *New York Times,* September 12, 2011, www.nytimes.com/2011/09/13/opinion/if-it-feelsright.html?scp=1&sq=%22If%20It%20Feels%20Right%22&st=cse.

3. Roffman, D. M. "Making Meaning and Finding Morality in a Sexualized World," in *Jewish Choices, Jewish Voices: Sex and Intimacy.* Edited by E. N. Dorff and Danya Ruttenberg. Philadelphia: Jewish Publication Society, 2010; Dorff, E. N. *This Is My Beloved, This Is My Friend: A Rabbinic Letter on Human Intimacy.* New York: Rabbinic Assembly, 1996.

4. Gold, T. "237 Reasons Why Women Have Sex." *The Guardian,* September 29, 2009, www.alternet.org/story/142952.

5. Douglas, S. *Enlightened Sexism: The Seductive Message that Feminism's Work Is Done.* New York: Times Books, 2010.

6. Dowd, M. "What's Up, Slut?" *New York Times,* July 16, 2006, page A25.

Chapter 7

1. Stepp, L. S. "Parents Are Alarmed by an Unsettling New Fad in Middle Schools: Oral Sex." *Washington Post,* July 8, 1999; Low, M. "Casual Sex Becomes Subject for Middle Schoolers." *Detroit Free Press,* June 11, 2002.

2. Radun, L. "Identifying and Setting Healthy Boundaries." www.youtube.com/watch?v=vWVA7J2sm6s.

3. Wallis, C. "What Makes Teens Tick." *Time,* September 26, 2008, www.time.com/time/magazine/article/0,9171,994126,00.html; Weinberger, D., B. Elvevag, and J. Gieed. *The Adolescent Brain: A Work in Progress.* Washington, DC: National Campaign to Prevent Teen

Pregnancy, June 2005; Baylin, J., and D. Hughes. "Brain-Based Parenting." *Psychotherapy Networker,* January/February 2012, pages 38–43, 56–57.

4. Wood, C. *Yardsticks: Children in the Classroom Ages 4–14.* Turners Falls, MA: Northeast Foundation for Children, 2007.

5. Flohr, D. "The Parent Circle." *Psychotherapy Networker,* January/February, 2012, pages 30–35, 54–55.

6. Berkowitz, A. "The Social Norms Approach: Theory, Research, and Annotated Bibliography." August 2004, www.alanberkowitz.com/articles/social_norms.pdf.

7. Lakoff, G. *Don't Think of an Elephant.* White River Junction, VT: Chelsea Green, 2004.

Chapter 8

1. Taffel, R. "The Decline and Fall of Parental Authority." *Psychotherapy Networker,* January /February 2012, pages 22–29, 52–55.

2. Ganeva, T. "How to Tart Up Your Infant: For a Start, Dress Them Up Like a Tiny Prostitute." AlterNet, November 28, 2008, www.alternet.org/blogs/sex/108898/11/21/08.

3. Henig, R. M. "The Post-Adolescent, Pre-Adult, Not-Quite-Decided Life Stage." *New York Times Magazine,* August 22, 2010, pages 28–37, 45–49.

4. Toomey, R. B., R. M. Diaz, and S. T. Russell. "High School Gay-Straight Alliances (GSAs) and Young Adult Well-Being: An Examination of GSA Presence, Participation, and Perceived Effectiveness." *Applied Developmental Science* 15, no. 4 (November 2011): 175–185; www.tandfonline.com/doi/full/10.1080/10888691.2011.607378.

5. Savin-Williams, R. C. *The New Gay Teenager.* Cambridge, MA: Harvard University Press, 2005; Brody, J. E. "Gay or Straight: Youths Aren't So Different." *New York Times,* January 4, 2011, page D7.

6. Huegel, K. *GLBT: The Survival Guide for Gay, Lesbian, Bisexual, Transgender, and Questioning Teens.* Minneapolis, MN: Free Spirit Publishing, 2011.

7. Jennings, K. *Always My Child: A Parent's Guide to Understanding Your Gay, Lesbian, Bisexual, Transgendered, or Questioning Son or Daughter.* New York: Fireside, 2003.

8. Ryan, C., and D. Futterman. *Lesbian and Gay Youth: Care and Counseling.* New York: Columbia University Press, 1998.

9. Bryan, J. *From the Dress-Up Corner to the Senior Prom: Navigating Gender and Sexuality Diversity in PreK–12 Schools.* New York: Rowman & Littlefield, 2012.

10. Klass, P. "Seeing Social Media More as Portal than as Pitfall." *New York Times,* January 10, 2012, page D5; Bazelon, E. "The Ninny State: The Dangers of Overprotecting Your Kids from Technology." *New York Times Magazine,* June 26, 2011, pages 11–12.

11. Bazelon, E. "The Young and the Friended: Why Facebook Is After Your Kids." *New York Times Magazine,* October 12, 2011, pages 15–16.

12. McCleese, J., and S. McCleese. "Seeking Balance: The Online Lives of Children." *Independent School Magazine,* Summer 2010.

13. Kaiser Family Foundation. "Media Multi-Tasking: Changing the Amount and Nature of Young People's Media Use." News release, March 9, 2005, www.kff.org/entmedia/entmedia 030905nr.cfm.

14. Delmonico, D., E. Griffin, and K. Edger. "Setting Limits in the Virtual World: Helping Families Develop Acceptable Use Policies." *Paradigm* 13, no. 4 (Fall 2008): 12–13, 22.

15. Fitzgerald, L. "Plastic Surgery Below the Belt." *Time,* November 19, 2008, www .time.com/time/health/article/0,8599,1859937,00.html.

16. Mitchell, K., D. Finkelhor, L. Jones, and J. Wolak. "Prevalence and Characteristics of Youth Sexting: A National Study." *Pediatrics* 129, no. 1 (January 1, 2012): 13–20; http://pediatrics.aappublications.org/content/129/1/13.full.

17. Hoffman, J. "A Girl's Nude Photo and Altered Lives." *New York Times Magazine,* March 26, 2011, www.nytimes.com/2011/03/27/us/27sexting.html?_r=1&scp=1&sq=A%20Girl%27s%20Nude%20Photo,%20and%20Altered%20Lives&st=cse.

18. Lithwick, D. "Teens, Nude Photos, and the Law." *Newsweek,* February 23, 2009, page 18.

Appendix

1. "Developing Healthy Communities: A Risk and Protective Factor Approach to Preventing Alcohol and Other Drug Abuse." Seattle: Developmental Research and Program, 1995.

2. Strauss, S. *Sexual Harassment and Teens: A Program for Positive Change.* Minneapolis, MN: Free Spirit, 1992.

3. "Dating Violence," a presentation by CHANA, a domestic violence educational service and prevention program sponsored by The Associated: Jewish Community Federation of Baltimore, Maryland.

Family Resources List

Books on Child and Adolescent Development

Brazelton, T. B. *Toddlers and Parents: A Declaration of Independence.* New York: Dell Publishing, 1989.

Brazelton, T. B., and Joshua D. Sparrow. *Touchpoints Three to Six: Your Child's Emotional and Behavioral Development.* Cambridge, MA: Da Capo Press, 2001.

Caissy, G. E. *Early Adolescence: Understanding the 10–15 Year Old.* Cambridge, MA: Da Capo Press, 1994.

Deak, J. *How Girls Thrive.* Da Capo Press. Green Blanket Press, 2010.

Elkind, D. *All Grown Up and No Place to Go.* Cambridge, MA: Da Capo Press, 1998.

Feinstein, S. *Parenting the Teenage Brain: A Work in Progress.* Lanham, MD: Rowman & Littlefield, 2009.

Fraiberg, S. H. *The Magic Years.* New York: Fireside, 1996.

Roffman, D. M. *"But How'd I Get in There in the First Place?": Talking to Your Young Child About Sex.* Cambridge, MA: Da Capo Press, 2002.

Sachs, B. *Emptying the Nest: Launching Your Young Adult Toward Success and Self-Reliance.* New York: Palgrave Macmillan, 2010.

———. *The Good Enough Child.* New York: HarperCollins, 2001.

———. *The Good Enough Teen.* New York: HarperCollins, 2005.

Thompson, M., and Catherine O'Neill-Grace. *Best Friends, Worst Enemies: Understanding the Social Lives of Children.* New York: Ballantine, 2002.

Thompson, M., and Teresa Barker. *It's a Boy!: Your Son's Development from Birth to 18.* New York: Ballantine, 2009.

Walsh, D. *WHY Do They Act That Way?: A Survival Guide to the Adolescent Brain for You and Your Teen.* New York: Free Press, 2005.

Wood, C. *Children in the Classroom Ages 4–14: A Resource for Parents and Teachers.* Turner Falls, MA: Northeast Foundation for Children, 2007.

See also www.gesellinstitute.org for individual books and pamphlets on child and early adolescent development, ages one through fourteen.

Additional Reading for Parents

Goleman, D. *Emotional Intelligence.* New York: Bantam Books, 1995.

Jennings, K. *Always My Child: A Parent's Guide to Understanding Your Gay, Lesbian, Bisexual, Transgendered, or Questioning Son or Daughter.* New York: Fireside, 2003.

Johnson, T. C. *Understanding Your Child's Sexual Behavior: What's Natural and Healthy.* Oakland, CA: New Harbinger Publications, 1999.

Kilbourne, J., and D. Levin. *So Sexy So Soon.* New York: Ballantine, 2009.

Kimmel, M. *Guyland: The Perilous World Where Boys Become Men.* New York: Harper, 2009.

Kindlon, D. *Too Much of a Good Thing: Raising Children of Character in an Indulgent Age.* New York: Hyperion, 2001.

Lamb, S., L. M. Brown, and Mark Tappan. *Packaging Boyhood*. New York: St. Martin's Press, 2009.

Orenstein, P. *Cinderella Ate My Daughter: Dispatches from the Front Lines of the New Girlie-Girl Culture*. New York: Harper, 2011.

Quart, A. *Branded*. Cambridge, MA: Da Capo Press, 2003.

Roffman, D. M. *Sex and Sensibility: The Thinking Parent's Guide to Talking Sense About Sex*. Cambridge, MA: Da Capo Press, 2001.

Sax, L. *Boys Adrift*. New York: Basic Books, 2007.

Taffle, R. *The Second Family: Dealing with Peer Power, Pop Culture, the Wall of Silence—and Other Challenges of Raising Today's Teens*. New York: St. Martin's Griffin, 2001.

Books for Young Children

These resources are considered some of the best in the field. You may want to check out these books and websites on your own first.

Bryan, J. *The Different Dragon*. Ridley Park, PA: Two Lives Publishing, 2006.

Cole, J. *How You Were Born*. New York: William Morrow, 1994.

Freeman, L. *It's My Body*. Seattle: Parenting Press, 1984.

Harris, R. *Happy Birth Day!* Somerville, MA: Candlewick, 2002.

———. *It's So Amazing!: A Book About Eggs, Sperm, Birth, Babies, and Families*. Somerville, MA: Candlewick, 2004.

———. *It's Not the Stork!: A Book About Girls, Boys, Babies, Bodies, Families, and Friends*. Somerville, MA: Candlewick, 2008.

Hindman, J., and Tom Novak. *A Very Touching Book . . . for Little People and Big People*. La Grande, OR: Alexandria Associates, 1983.

Kilodavis, C. *My Princess Boy*. New York: Simon & Schuster, 2011.

Newman, L. *Heather Has Two Mommies*. Los Angeles: Alyson Publications, 2000.

———. *Mommy, Momma, and Me*. New York: First Tricycle Press, 2009.

Parr, T. *The Family Book*. New York: Little, Brown Books, 2010.

Richardson, J., and Peter Parnell. *And Tango Makes Three*. New York: Simon & Schuster, 2005.

Schoen, M. *Belly Buttons Are Navels*. New York: Prometheus, 1990.

Willhoite, M. *Daddy's Roommate*. Los Angeles: Alyson Publications, 1990.

Books for Late Elementary/Middle School Children

Gitchel, S., and Lorri Foster. *Let's Talk About S-E-X: A Guide for Kids 9–12 and Their Parents*. Deephaven, MN: Book Peddlers, 2005.

Gravelle, K. *The Period Book*. New York: Walker and Company, 2006.

———. *What's Going on Down There?: Answers to Questions Boys Find Hard to Ask*. New York: Walker and Company, 1998.

Harris, R. *It's Perfectly Normal: Changing Bodies, Growing Up, Sex, and Sexual Health*. Somerville, MA: Candlewick Publishing, 2009.

Middleman, A. *American Medical Association Boy's Guide to Becoming a Teen*. San Francisco: Jossey-Bass, 2006.

Schaefer, V. L. *Care and Keeping of You: The Body Book for Girls*. Middleton, WI: American Girl Library, 1998.

See also: multiple books by Linda Madaras and Area Madaras, for boys and girls: www.new marketpress.org.

Books for High School–Age Children

Basso, M. J. *The Underground Guide to Teenage Sexuality.* Minneapolis, MN: Fairview Press, 2003.

Bell, R. *Changing Bodies, Changing Lives: A Book for Teens on Sex and Relationships.* New York: Random House, 1998.

Corinna, H. *S.E.X.: The All-You-Need-to-Know Progressive Sexuality Guide to Get You Through High School and College.* New York: Marlowe and Company, 2007.

Columbia University's Health Education Program. *The "Go Ask Alice" Book of Answers: A Guide to Good Physical, Sexual and Emotional Health.* New York: Holt Paperbacks, 1998.

Huegel, K. *GLBTQ: The Survival Guide for Gay, Lesbian, Bisexual, Transgender, and Questioning Teens.* Minneapolis, MN: Free Spirit Publishing, 2011.

See also sexetc.org and www.scarleteen.com.

Helpful Websites: Parents Talking to Kids About Sexuality

Advocates for Youth: www.advocatesforyouth.org

Answer: www.answer.rutgers.edu

Parents, Families, and Friends of Lesbians and Gays: www.pflag.org

Planned Parenthood: www.plannedparenthood.org

Sexuality Information and Education Council of the United States: www.siecus.org

Helpful Websites: Internet Safety

Childnet International: www.childnet-int.org

Connect Safely: www.connectsafely.org

CyberSMART: www.cybersmart.org

Family Online Safety Institute: www.fosi.org

FilterReview: www.filterreview.com

SafeKids: www.safekids.com/kidsrules.htm

Appendix:
Some Basic Facts
All Adults Should Know

Organs, Systems, and Openings

In my teaching I'm constantly amazed at how little children and teens know about the bodies they inhabit. It would be wonderful if adults were to begin teaching children "body basics" very deliberately when they are very young. The process begins, of course, with labeling the body parts they can see, touch, and experience directly, and it's good policy to name their sexual parts with the same matter-of-fact tone and terminology. As children approach age three or four, we can also begin to educate them about the fact that bodies have an *inside* and an *outside,* and that many of our parts—or organs— are located where we can't see them. An easy way to teach this concept is by helping children understand what happens to their food after they swallow it and can't see it anymore. (There are many clever and engaging big-picture books available in stores and public libraries that show and educate younger children about the internal parts of the body.)

Gradually we'll also be able to explain that each organ inside our body is connected to other organs and that, together, certain groups of organs make up each of our various body systems. We have many different body systems, and in each one a group of different organs works together to do a specific job that helps keep our body alive and healthy. Once children have grasped this larger concept, we'll be in a good position eventually to fit the reproductive system, literally, right into the body along with all the others—making it ever so much easier to talk and learn about because there will be already be a ready-made context. The conversation won't be about SEX! but simply a continuation of many earlier low-key and matter-of-fact discussions about how our bodies work.

Another really important concept to teach young children about is *body openings* (it's much clearer to say "openings" instead of "holes"): We have several places on the *outside* of our bodies that lead to specific places on the *inside*. It's through these openings that things *from the outside go into* our bodies, and other things *from the inside go out*. With very little effort, adults can use all kinds of everyday experiences to reinforce those ideas very concretely. These basic anatomical concepts are important for children to grasp in a general way, and they will also provide a ready-made context for explaining the mechanics of intercourse and birth later on.

Be sure to explain eventually as well that girls and women have *three* of these openings in the area between their legs—the urinary, vaginal, and anal openings—and that these openings are connected to tubes, organs, and systems (urinary, reproductive, and digestive) that are *not connected to each other either structurally or functionally*. When we're not clear about those distinctions, most kids surmise that these three systems are somehow all blended together. Without very skilled teaching, that conclusion will be hard for them to "unlearn" later; many teens and adult women and men even today are still under the impression that women urinate through their vaginas.

Stomachs, Abdomens, and Uteruses

Food and stomachs are very real to children and easy for them to understand. Unless we're very careful in how we speak to them when they are young, most grow up thinking that their stomach, their belly or abdomen, and their abdominal wall are one and the same. This sloppy terminology—especially if we also tell children at some point that babies grow in stomachs or bellies—sets them up for untold confusion later on.

Vaginas and Vulvas

An even more fundamental confusion exists about the female genitals. The vulva is the collective name for all of the *external* female genitalia, which include the inner and outer labia (or vaginal "lips"), the clitoris, and the mons (the mound of skin on top of the pubic bone where pubic hair eventually grows). The vagina, contrary to popular opinion, is not located, even partially, on the outside of the female anatomy. The vagina is an internal pouch—

actually best thought of as a "collapsed" space located just inside the vaginal opening, kind of like the finger of a glove with no finger in it; when there's nothing inside of a vagina, its walls are touching. Thinking that the vagina is located somewhere on the outside or that it is both inside *and* outside, as many people do, is tantamount to not knowing the difference between your face and your throat!

Another topic to explain with great care is the hymen, a typically thin and fairly flexible piece of skin or tissue located just inside the vagina that *partially* blocks its opening (otherwise it would impede the menstrual flow). It is present in most but not all baby girls. Some hymens disappear naturally in the process of maturation—it has no physiological purpose—or as a result of activities such as gymnastics or other forms of exercise. Therefore, the absence of a hymen in no way proves that a girl or woman has experienced vaginal intercourse, though its presence likely means she hasn't.

The language associated with what happens to hymens at first intercourse— that it pops, tears, rips, breaks, etc.—is unnecessarily scary and misleading. Here's how I like to explain it: Almost all hymens have one or more openings that are usually pretty flexible. If something larger than the opening goes through it—a tampon, for example—the opening will become bigger, and bigger still as the tampon is removed because it will likely be wider. If a penis goes through the opening, the opening will become so wide that the hymen will no longer exist as a barrier. As a result, there may be discomfort, sometimes to the point of pain, and/or a little bit of blood may appear, since a small piece of skin is being separated from the vaginal wall. Afterward the girl or woman may feel some soreness, which may also reoccur the next couple of times she has intercourse.

Pain or discomfort with first intercourse (or any) is actually more likely to result from a lack of vaginal lubrication or tenseness in the strong muscles that surround the opening of the vagina than the presence of the hymen. Gentleness, and a caring relationship with someone who understands female anatomy and sexual response—along with learning how to relax the vaginal muscles and using a commercially available lubricant, such as K-Y jelly—can help the process enormously. (Girls and women can demonstrate to themselves that they can deliberately tense and relax these muscles—the same ones they use to stop and start the flow of urine—at will. Tensing and relaxing them during a sexual experience can also heighten sexual pleasure.) It's important to know, too, that although tenseness and lack of lubrication may result from the newness of the situation, they may also be a sign that the person is not feeling ready enough, or trusting enough, or aroused enough to participate in intercourse. Our bodies are wise and tell us important things about our emotional state that we would be wise to heed. As someone I know once said, "Sexual intercourse is never an emergency."

Males Have Reproductive Parts, Too

Even today the children and adolescents I teach—both girls and boys—are often incredibly confused about such basic concepts as the difference between sperm and semen, or erections and ejaculations. And the terms "vas deferens," "seminal vesicle," and "prostate gland" aren't even in their memory banks.

Here are some basics: Testicles, or testes, located in a sac behind the penis, are the male gonads (the female gonads are the ovaries). They make the male hormone, testosterone, responsible for creating the body changes that occur during pubescence, and also for the ongoing production of sperm after puberty. (Estrogen, the female sex hormone, serves exactly parallel functions: stimulating the body changes during pubescence, and playing a central role in the female menstrual cycle going forward.) As sperm leave the testicles, they enter the sperm ducts or vas deferens, two tubes that carry the sperm into the body (analogous to the fallopian tubes, or oviducts, in the female, into which eggs pass after ovulation) and toward two semen-producing organs known as the seminal vesicles.

Eventually the two sperm ducts join with a third tube from the bladder (the urethra) inside the prostate gland, creating one tube that passes through the penis. It's at this point that the urinary and reproductive systems join in the male body. The prostate gland makes an additional part of the semen, and, at the point of ejaculation, mixes the sperm and semen together and helps pump the mixture out through the penis in a series of spurts. Boys, quite logically, often want to know whether urination and ejaculation can happen at the same time; since the muscle at the base of the bladder contracts whenever a firm erection occurs, it's not possible for that to happen. It's also important for boys to understand that erections are the result of increased blood flow to the "spongy" tissues (yup, that's what they're called) of the penis, and that erections can happen for a variety of reasons—sometimes at unexpected times and places—especially during pubescence. Most erections simply go away, as the muscles surrounding the blood vessels relax; in a sexual situation where ejaculation occurs, the penis will begin to soften soon thereafter.

Puberty, Pubescence, and Hormones

In common usage, the word "puberty" has two very different meanings: (1) the specific body changes (secondary sex characteristics) children undergo as their bodies develop and mature from girl to woman, or boy to man; (2) the point in time when boys and girls become fertile. I much prefer to separate the two meanings—by using the word "pubescence" to refer to the former and "puberty" the latter—because it helps kids to better understand their own development. The changes associated with pubescence occur very gradually over many years, starting internally at about the age of eight, and ending when young women and men achieve their full adult height. Puberty, on the other hand, is the *point in time* when a boy or girl becomes reproductively capable, an event marked either by a girl's first period or a boy's first ejaculation. For most young people, these two experiences happen long before the process of pubescence is complete, but are nonetheless important to highlight because from this moment on creating a pregnancy is possible. Moreover, what *all* kids in this stage have in common is that they are "pubescing" a little bit more every single day; exactly when each one of them will reach puberty is highly variable, and can be as young as eight and as old as eighteen. That helps "early" or "late" developers feel they are more like their peers than different.

Here's the definition of hormones I drill into my seventh-grade (and older) students: "A hormone is a chemical messenger that's made in one part of the body, travels through the bloodstream to another part of the body, and tells it what to do." Everything reproductive that occurs in the body, and all of the body changes during pubescence, result from hormonal messages from the brain and gonads. Though fluctuating hormones are a fact of life for teens and many preteens, here's a caution about using the word in regard to their behavior: Even though hormone changes can affect mood, and moods can influence behavior, normal, healthy teenagers are capable of controlling their behavior (including sexual behavior) at all times. Talking about adolescents as if they are driven by "raging hormones" may imply otherwise, just at a point in their development when we most need to reinforce the importance of personal responsibility.

Wet Dreams or Nocturnal Emissions

Though wet dreams are definitely *wet,* I wish we could deemphasize the "dream" part. Adults often tell boys that wet dreams happen because a boy has a sexy dream. Wet dreams happen because the body has a storage issue! There's too much accumulated sperm and semen in the tubes and organs, and a wet dream is the body's way of making room for more. (If boys begin to have ejaculations when they're awake, their periodic wet dreams will stop.) Wet dreams happen during the REM-sleep part of the sleep cycle, when, conveniently, penises are already erect, but a boy may or may not remember the dream, and it may or may not have been sexual in nature. Though it's certainly true that a wet dream can be a profound and very pleasurable sexual experience for a boy—and a great opening for talking about such matters—I worry that some boys may hesitate to come talk to us or ask questions in the first place if they think doing so amounts to an "admission" they've been having "sex dreams." By the way, some boys don't have wet dreams, and that's normal, too. (And some sexually inactive men do.)

Of course, all of the above information is important and appropriate for both boys and girls to know and understand. Demystifying these processes for everyone is exactly the point.

Menstrual Periods and Menstrual Cycles

In helping girls and boys understand what periods are all about, it's very helpful to first explain why there is a blood lining in the uterus in the first place, since that helps them make sense of why it comes out. Since fetuses don't breathe or eat while in the uterus, they need to receive oxygen and nutrition directly from their mother's bloodstream. This transfer is accomplished by the round, flat pregnancy organ called the placenta that is attached on one side to the inside of the uterus, where there are lots of blood vessels, and on the other side to the fetus's umbilical cord. During pregnancy, fetal blood comes through the cord to the placenta and picks up oxygen and nutrition directly from the mother's bloodstream. The oxygen- and nutrition-rich fetal blood goes back to the fetus and flows directly into its bloodstream (no stomach or lungs needed). During a menstrual cycle when no pregnancy has been created, the uterus eventually receives a hormonal message to send the lining out since it is not needed.

Kids, and many adults, too, are often mighty confused about the workings of the female menstrual cycle, and even about the difference between a menstrual *cycle* and a menstrual *period*. The most important starting place is to explain that the menstrual cycle is a series of reproductive events that occur in a girl's or woman's body, every twenty-eight days on average. The menstrual period (the shedding of the lining) is only *one* event in the series. Others include: rebuilding of the uterine lining, release of the egg from an ovary, death of the egg, secretion of nourishment into the uterine lining, and recognition by the ovaries that there's no pregnancy this cycle. (Notice that the egg dies and disintegrates *many days before* the lining is released; the egg doesn't come out with the lining.) In keeping track of the cycle, it's important to know that each new cycle *begins* on the first day of the menstrual period: "Day one" of the cycle equals "day one" of the period. This date, known as the LMP, for the first day of the last menstrual period, is what all girls and women should check on their calendar each time a new cycle begins.

The risk of becoming pregnant over the course of any given menstrual cycle is also a confusing concept. Here's the way I like to explain it: Because the timing of so many events in the cycle is variable, there are no times during the menstrual cycle when pregnancy can be ruled out entirely; there are no absolutely "safe times," only relatively less or more *unsafe* times. What that means is that people who definitely want to avoid a pregnancy must either abstain from sexual intercourse or use an approved method of contraception consistently and correctly each and every time it's needed.

Information for Parents (and Teens) About Prevention
In recent decades, "prevention science" researchers have studied specific "risk" and "protective" factors that affect the incidence of risk-taking behaviors

among adolescents. Risk factors are those conditions that statistically *increase* a young person's chances of engaging in problem behaviors, such as premature or unprotected sexual behavior, or alcohol and other drug use. Protective factors, on the other hand, create conditions that *decrease* the probability of engaging in potentially risky behaviors.[1]

This research is a gift to you as a parent, for a host of reasons. Most important, it identifies multiple strategies for setting up the conditions that support your children in making healthy choices. It demonstrates that you can strongly and positively influence your children's decisions, by *minimizing* the risk factors present in their world, and *maximizing* the protective factors. Recognizing that as a parent you have in your power that kind of potential impact can be a vital confidence booster, especially during the teen years when your children are increasingly out and about in the world, beyond your direct reach.

As you'll see, what parents need to do is all pretty standard stuff, and not surprisingly, it's all about wearing your "suit" and staying the course. What's more, these same strategies also reduce the incidence of a variety of serious problem behaviors among adolescents, including delinquency, school dropout, and violence. They are *that* powerful.

The data from these studies is clear: what makes the biggest difference in children and teens engaging in healthy versus unhealthy decision-making is the experience of "connectedness"—primarily at home, but also at school and other places. So, yes, placing a priority on having dinner as a family two to three times a week, and students' feeling that teachers care about them as individuals, do make a real difference. Regardless of the situations in which they may find themselves, having these kinds of strong bonds with important adults and institutions in their lives appears to fortify their ability to make good and healthy decisions. It is a form of protection they take with them wherever they go.

According to the research findings, here are the specific kinds of conditions that matter for kids in reducing their level of risk:

- Close relationships with parents and other family members
- Success in school

- ✓ Meaningful connections to "pro-social" institutions (such as school, religious groups, service groups, etc.)
- ✓ Parents who communicate clear standards and expectations
- ✓ Parents who follow through with close monitoring of where their children are, who they are with, and what kind of supervision is in place

Conversely, among the factors that put young people at *greater risk* for problem behaviors are the following:

- ✓ Ineffective or inconsistent parenting
- ✓ Weak school performance
- ✓ Associating with peers who engage in risky behaviors
- ✓ Overestimating the number of peers who engage in risky behaviors (see the information on normative-belief research in Chapter 7)
- ✓ Poor social coping skills

Nothing is a guarantee either way, of course. But it's certainly a gift to have such pointed scientific knowledge at our disposal to tell us what's most important to beware of, strengthen, and watch out for.

How to Teach Your Teenager as Little as Possible

Even now I still have an occasional nightmare about taking a test in high school or college. I was never confident I'd studied enough, mostly because teachers were always trying to cram into our heads as much information as possible.

Becoming a health educator was a welcome relief. In my field the goal is just the opposite: to teach as little as possible—over and over and in different ways—so students will be able to remember, store, and use it well as needed. Here are some ways to teach your kids as little as possible about some important prevention topics.

Talking About Pregnancy Prevention

The number and types of contraceptives (temporary methods of birth control) available today is truly mind-boggling. The best way to think about and teach about a long list of *anything* is to organize the examples into categories: Some methods of contraception are available over-the-counter in pharmacies and many supermarkets; for others, a doctor's visit and a prescription are required. Some work by keeping the sperm from getting to the egg, some keep the egg in the ovary so it can't meet up with a sperm, and others prevent implantation. Many types of contraception for women contain hormones, but they differ in the way the hormones enter the person's bloodstream. Some kinds of contraception are very effective, if always used consistently and correctly, while others aren't very effective even if all instructions are followed perfectly. Making these kinds of distinctions helps everyone understand what's important to know and think about regarding this complicated subject. Giving a long list of examples and specific information about each isn't nearly as helpful, or as memorable, from a practical standpoint.

Parents should not hesitate to talk to their children at any age about contraception if they ask about it. (In my view, the best time for parents to initiate the conversation with basic concepts is in late elementary school.) Contraception is simply another interesting topic to know about in life. Their curiosity about it means little or nothing about their immediate need for it, and our telling about it doesn't mean we think they need it.

Sometimes parents ask whether they should provide condoms (for preventing disease and/or pregnancy) or other forms of contraception for their children. That's an individual family decision that depends on many variables. As a general rule, I favor an approach where young people understand that sexual intercourse is grown-up behavior that requires a grown-up level of responsibility, including acquiring and using any prevention required. I would also be concerned if parents project an "Oh well, I guess you're going to do it anyway" message.

Talking About Sexually Transmitted Infections (STIs)

STD ("D" for disease) or STI ("I" for infection) are the most commonly used terms for sexually transmitted diseases or infections. I prefer the latter because it puts the emphasis on germs, not on disease. Most people who suffer from STIs don't look diseased and may not even know they're infected.

Something I really believe is that the average person probably can't remember more than three things—unless she uses the information on a regular basis—for any great length of time. So, in my teaching, I'm always trying to boil things down to "threes."

Since there are at least six different sexually transmitted infections that are really important to know about, we're already in trouble. Here are some interesting and informative ways to think and talk about these infections, almost all in "threes":

- ✓ Three of the six most common STIs—syphilis, gonorrhea, and chlamydia—are bacterial infections, which means they can be cured with antibiotic drugs (though the person may be left with body damage that may or may not be reversible).
- ✓ Three of the six most common STIs—HIV/AIDS, genital herpes, and HPV/genital warts—are viral infections. Antibiotic drugs don't work against viruses, so doctors generally can't cure them. They can treat only the symptoms and long-term effects of these infections on the body.
- ✓ Two of these infections—syphilis and HIV—are potentially life threatening, because the germs make their way to the bloodstream and can dangerously affect vital organ systems. These two infections can also be spread in nonsexual ways, through direct blood-to-blood contact.
- ✓ The remaining four (sorry) infections—chlamydia, gonorrhea, herpes, and HPV/genital warts—generally stay put in a person's sexual and reproductive organs, where they don't cause life-threatening damage. (Untreated gonorrhea and chlamydia, which act very similarly in the body, can cause serious fertility problems.) The one exception is that women with a history of HPV or genital herpes infections are at higher risk for cancer of the cervix, which if untreated may in fact become life threatening.
- ✓ Three kinds of sexual behaviors can lead to the spread of sexually transmitted infections: genital-to-genital, genital-to-mouth, and genital-to-anal contact with an infected partner.
- ✓ There are three direct ways to prevent the spread of STI germs: abstaining from the three behaviors above; engaging in a completely monogamous relationship (two people who *never* engage in these

behaviors with anyone but each other are in a closed system); and using a male or female condom, which creates a barrier between body parts so the germs won't spread (very effective, if used consistently and correctly, but not perfectly so).

✓ There are three steps to using a male latex condom correctly: (1) It must be put in place *before* the above body parts are in contact, and *after* the penis is erect. (2) It's unrolled onto the penis down to the base, with air-free space left at the tip (accomplished by squeezing) to catch the ejaculate. (3) The penis must be removed from the other person's body very soon after ejaculation (because the penis will lose its erection and the condom will slip off), with fingers held around it to hold the condom in place.

No matter how you slice and dice it, STIs are a complicated subject. But although the six infections differ from one another in important ways, from the perspective of prevention, *all of them* have two essential things in common: they're all transmitted through the exact same sexual behaviors, and they're all prevented in the exact same ways. That simplifies things a lot.

A final area of confusion for many kids and adults is the difference between pregnancy prevention and STI prevention. When a couple is trying to prevent a pregnancy, their goal is to keep an egg and sperm from touching (or a fertilized egg away from the uterine wall); in preventing the spread of infection, the goal is to keep one body part from touching another part that may be infected. These are two very different propositions, but because condoms can accomplish both of those goals, many teens who don't receive adequate instruction assume that all methods of pregnancy prevention also prevent the spread of infection.

Talking About Date/Acquaintance Rape

We have a long, sad history in American culture of blaming rape victims for their own rapes. For quite a while, after so-called rape shield laws were passed in the United States, prohibiting defense attorneys from asking alleged victims about their sexual history in the courtroom to discredit them, I noticed a decided change in attitudes. Among adults, and my students as well, I rarely heard anyone claim or even infer that girls and women got raped because they "asked for it." More recently I've begun to hear those kinds of attitudes creeping back into classroom discussion, even among girls. I fear that rape-themed pornography, so accessible today, may be a contributing factor, and also that endless exposure to images that constantly reduce women to mere stereotypes or objects has eroded some people's capacity for empathy. I also fear that girls who are victimized will themselves buy into this belief system, blame themselves for what happened, and not seek the help they need to get past it.

Parents and teachers need to give very straight messages to boys and girls. There is only one cause of rape, and it is *the decision in the mind of the rapist* to overrule another person's basic needs and rights and overtake her (or his) body in a horrific way.

That said, we can also help our children be smart about the risk and protective factors that can increase or decrease the chance that they will be targeted for sexual assault—or wrongly accused of committing it. I will list way more than three. The more strategies they know for minimizing their own risk factors and maximizing their protective factors, the safer they will be.

One final thought: It's very important to impress upon teens that even if they are careless or reckless, and do the opposite of the things on the list above, they are still *absolutely not responsible* for someone's decision to take advantage of their poor judgment. No matter how many poor choices they may have made, none of them is *ever* even in the same ballpark as a rapist's decision to rape.

Here are some common risk and protective factors that can increase or decrease the chance that a young person may be targeted for rape. Note that none of the risk factors listed is *a cause* of rape; rape can and does occur when none of these factors are present.

Risk Factors

- Use of alcohol or other drugs by the victim and/or rapist
- Prematurely trusting another person's intentions, and agreeing to be alone

- ✓ Going to a party alone when most or all of the people there are not well known to you, especially if they are older and more socially experienced
- ✓ Being overconfident; assuming, without thinking things through, that a particular person or location is safe
- ✓ Dressing or acting in a sexualized way (this, like all of the others, is *not* a cause, but it may attract unwanted attention)
- ✓ Lack of assertiveness, which may lead to "going along" in circumstances where your gut tells you it's not what you want, or that things just don't feel right

Protective Factors

- ✓ Always being with at least one person you know well, who stays sober, and agreeing to watch out for each other's safety
- ✓ Understanding that trust is *always* earned. Most people are kind at heart and won't hurt you, but knowing that a person is genuinely trustworthy requires a track record.
- ✓ Drinking only out of closed beverage containers in a party situation, to avoid consuming "date rape" or other drugs. If you put a drink down and take your eyes off it even for a moment, *always* throw it out and get a new one.
- ✓ Being knowledgeable about the effects of even a small quantity of alcohol or other drugs on your body and thought processes
- ✓ Having a "no questions asked until tomorrow" agreement with parents or another adult that they will immediately come pick you up at any time from anywhere, even if you've lied about your whereabouts or activities, with no conversation until the next day
- ✓ Carrying a fully charged cell phone whenever you go out

Talking About Sexual Harassment

Sexual harassment is a unique form of bullying. Legally it refers to "uninvited, unwanted, or unwelcome" sexual attention directed toward an individual in a school or workplace that is "persistent, pervasive, or severe."[2]

Between a superior and subordinate it is an abuse of real power; between peers in a school environment, it is a particularly effective way of gaining social power by making others feel small, helpless, "less than," and inferior. Left unchecked, it can have severe emotional, physical, social, and/or academic consequences for boys and girls who are targeted.

Sexually harassing behaviors in a school environment can take many forms and do not have to be physical in nature: verbal comments about parts of the body, clothing, the way a person looks, or sexual acts; spreading sexual rumors or name-calling; sending unwanted sexual content via cell, e-mail, texting, or any other kind of electronic media; leers, stares, and other facial expressions of a sexual nature; gestures with the hands or body; pressure for sexual activity; cornering or blocking; pulling at clothes; graffiti; howling, catcalls, or whistles; any unwanted touching of another person's sexual parts (which would also be a form of sexual assault). Some young people engage in these behaviors out of ignorance, inexperience, or "cluelessness," and once the effect on the other person is brought to their attention, they apologize and stop. If the behavior is truly intended to harass, it will likely continue until adults become involved and take the steps necessary to make certain that it ceases. Persistent sexual harassment, or any other kind of bullying or harassment, needs to be taken very seriously. It's never just a matter of "kids being kids."

Talking About Abusive Relationships

As much as we might not want to believe it, thousands and thousands of teenagers on any given day are caught up in abusive romantic and sexual relationships. Like domestic abuse, these experiences can leave deep emotional scars and may result in physical violence. One important thing parents can do by way of prevention is make sure their children, from an early age, can easily identify the characteristics of both healthy and unhealthy relationships. In an ongoing way, we can help children identify and verbalize what makes them—and other people—feel good and happy at certain times in certain relationships, and feel confused, angry, sad, or hurt in others. Drawing connections for them between healthy relationships and the core values addressed in Chapter 6—such as respect, trust, caring, loyalty, fairness, and equality—will help them size up all kinds of situations. Most important of all, children and teens who feel fundamentally good about themselves, and who have strong interpersonal skills, are much less likely to allow themselves to be mistreated.

Here are some warning signs of abusive relationships that we and especially our teenage children need to be aware of. They are excerpted from an excellent presentation on abusive relationships[3] my students recently viewed:

- Extreme jealousy
- Constant belittling and put-downs
- Ridiculing the other person in front of peers
- Telling the other person what to do
- Explosive bouts of temper
- Verbal threats
- Preventing the other person from doing what she or he wants to do
- Isolating the other person from friends and family
- Calling, e-mailing, and/or texting every few minutes to check on where the person is and what he or she is doing
- Checking the other person's computer or cell phone to see with whom he or she has been in contact
- Any kind of physical violence, including scratching, pushing, punching, biting, kicking, throwing objects, holding someone down, slapping, etc.
- Any kind of unwanted sexual touching or pressure

Index